Essentials of Private Practice

More Advance Acclaim for *Essentials of Private Practice*

"Dr. Hunt's work is an outstanding guide for running a successful private practice. Expertly combining business savvy with sound clinical common sense, Hunt draws from her rich repertoire of professional experience in order to show how sound clinical principles lead to an efficient private practice. *Essentials of Private Practice* is an essential resource and should have a place in every practitioner's library."

> —Concepcion Barrio, Ph.D., Associate Professor, San Diego State University School of Social Work

"Dr. Hunt offers much needed practical information on how to run the business side of a mental health practice in order to maximize profit and reduce stress. This highly useful material is not usually provided in graduate courses. The new as well as the seasoned private practitioner will find this a helpful guide."

> —Sandra Levy Ceren, Ph.D., Diplomate, American Board of Family Psychology

"Dr. Hunt's book is an indispensable resource for beginning independent practitioners. Having *Essentials of Private Practice* on your bookshelf is like having a professional consultant on call! Established practitioners will also benefit from studying and implementing Dr. Hunt's excellent ideas for reducing costs and stress while enhancing income."

> —Jana N. Martin, Ph.D., Licensed Psychologist and Past President of the California Psychological Association

A NORTON PROFESSIONAL BOOK

Essentials of Private Practice
Streamlining Costs, Procedures, and Policies for Less Stress

Holly A. Hunt

W. W. Norton & Company
New York • London

Copyright © 2005 by Holly A. Hunt

For information about permission to reproduce selections from this book, write to
Permissions, W. W. Norton & Company, Inc., 500 Fifth Avenue, New York, NY 10110

Production Manager: Leeann Graham
Manufacturing by R. R. Donnelly–Harrisonburg

Library of Congress Cataloging-in-Publication Data

Hunt, Holly A.
Essentials of private practice : streamlining costs, procedures, and policies for less stress /
Holly A. Hunt.
    p.   cm.
"A Norton professional book."
Includes index.
ISBN 0-393-70448-3 (pbk.)
1. Medicine—Practice 2. Medicine—Practice—Management. 3. Medical offices—Finance.
I. Title.

R728.H823 2004
610'.68—dc22   2004052078

W. W. Norton & Company, Inc., 500 Fifth Avenue, New York, N.Y. 10110
www.wwnorton.com

W. W. Norton & Company Ltd., Castle House, 75/76 Wells St., London W1T 3QT

    3   5   7   9   0   8   6   4   2

To my grandmother, Dorothy S. Hunt, the first and the best businesswoman I've ever known.

Contents

Appendices

Preface

Are you planning to be or already in private practice? I decided to write this book to share some strategies that have worked for me over the years in the hopes that they will help you too. The following chapters offer practical ways to streamline your practice by increasing day-to-day efficiency and eliminating unnecessary costs. Whether you are just starting out or have been at it awhile, these steps aim to help you thrive in your business so you can do the therapy work you want as long as you choose. They have worked so well for me that I can now support myself seeing clients one to two days a week.

If you find yourself in any of the following circumstances, this book may be especially appealing to you: Are you in graduate school and already dreaming about having your own practice? Are you newly-licensed and ready to be your own boss soon? Are you are already working hard in someone else's practice that reaps a healthy profit while your compensation is much less? I've been there, too. After joining my first group practice when I became licensed, I realized the financial agreement would quickly lead to a diminishing return for me. Although self-employed, I still paid a tiered percentage of income to the group. Even though my percentage rose the more I made, I figured that I would be making much more if I left the group.

Perhaps you are working more hours and feeling more tension in your own practice, but your take-home pay seems to be shrinking instead of growing. Count me in on this one, too. After eight months I left my first group and joined others in different expense-sharing arrangements for the next ten years. I definitely felt more pressure and less pay during these years, as managed care pushed out higher paying indemnity and PPO (preferred provider organization) insurance, panels began to close, and contracted fees were regularly slashed. More non-paid work was added, too, including treatment reports, case reviews, and special billing instructions for different managed care companies. Client stressors added to the mix, things such as no-shows, last-minute cancellations, and calls at all hours.

Perhaps you have a busy practice and are ready to scale down to pursue other interests, but still need to earn enough to pay your bills. I'm right with you on this one as well. After ten years of expense sharing with others, I moved to an office by myself where I have been ever since. I decided to reduce my practice hours so I could write this book, but, I still needed to earn enough to support myself.

The strategies in this book emerged from these years of different practice arrangements and assorted trials and tribulations. I pass them along to you as your colleague and ally, right beside you in the trenches of daily practice, hopefully saving you time and frustration in your own efforts.

The good news is that regardless of your current circumstances, you can have the practice you want with less stress and more income. The following chapters emphasize three main strategies to achieve these practice goals: lowering overhead expenses, simplifying daily procedures, and implementing efficient client policies. These organizational and business aspects of our work can be easily overlooked, but are crucial to a successful practice.

If you are in graduate school, you probably already have a good idea how to conduct therapy based on experiences in your classes, practicum, or internship. However, you may not have much familiarity with the business of private practice. Although there are many resources available that focus on the therapeutic side of our work, there are fewer devoted to setting up and operating our private practices.

If you are just beginning or already have a practice, you may not know where to go for assistance in your efforts. When I was starting out, I had no business training and did not know how to set up an office or develop daily procedures and policies. It was a daunting task to blend hard business matters with the caring and therapeutic approach inherent to psychotherapy.

This book aims to fill this gap and, in so doing, offer you a practice management resource. It is written directly for you, with your unique, dual status as both therapist and proprietor in mind. You will gain knowledge and skills about how to blend both of these roles, lower your strain, and increase your financial return within your daily practice. Your clients will also benefit from your increasingly well-run practice.

Private practice has definitely changed over the years, with economic concerns more dominant now than ever before. If you are a new practitioner, you enter a world in which most of the insured population is covered by some form of managed care. If you are an established practitioner, you have probably experienced the reduction of therapy fees while your overhead expenses have remained constant or have increased.

Many in practice have responded by increasing client loads to compensate for lowered rates. Others have added marketing efforts geared towards the self-pay population. While both of these strategies can be effective, they do require money, time, effort, and can become an increased burden to you. Consider also that when you are in need of more income, your prospective clients are likely to be struggling too. They may forgo self-pay therapy when basic expenses like mortgage, food, and clothes become a priority. This climate leads to more therapists competing for fewer and fewer cash-pay clients, creating more marketing work for you with less potential return on your time and energy investment.

This book presents other alternative methods to preserve and expand your income through cutting costs and improving efficiency. Whether you market a little or a lot, whether you desire a small or large practice, these strategies can make your work easier while actually increasing take-home pay. They will allow you to see managed care clients if you choose to and still earn a good income. By retaining a base level of income in the lean times, you will add a layer of protection during any unexpected shifts in client loads. You will also boost quality care to clients, enhancing rather than detracting from the therapeutic process and outcome.

As you read the chapters that follow, please note that to preserve confidentiality, I've changed client and practitioner names as well as identifying information. The first major streamlining strategy of reducing overhead expenses is covered in Chapters 1 through 3. Since we are often less knowledgeable about the business part of our work, we can easily lose potential profits through unchecked expenditures. You will learn ways to cut costs when arranging your practice, selecting your office, and choosing a communications system. By designing your practice with lower overhead in mind, you can ensure savings and increased earnings independent of your client load.

The second major strategy of this book involves streamlining routine procedures. Many clinicians in practice lose time, energy, and income through disorganized daily operations. Chapters 4 through 6 will help you simplify daily procedures to prevent these drains. You will learn how to efficiently arrange for initial appointments, verify insurance benefits, bill insurance carriers, and get paid quickly. These suggestions will help maximize your pay with minimal effort, allowing you to provide higher quality care to clients. Although my recommendations have you in mind as the person performing these daily operations, if you decide to have someone else do any of these services, you can also adapt this information to use in training your support staff.

The third major strategy involves implementing efficient client policies. Most of us enter this field with a primary desire to offer therapeutic services. We are typically sensitive, empathic, and intuitive, with much to offer as healers. These very qualities also make us vulnerable to exhaustion from the rigorous emotional needs of our clients. Chapters 7 through 9 will guide you in preserving your therapeutic gifts by establishing firm and caring policies—policies that will help both your clients and you at the same time. You will learn how to manage your finances wisely and efficiently collect the client fees you earn. You will read how to create and implement a successful cancellation policy to minimize violations and preserve your income if they do occur. You will also learn effective phone practices and policies to enhance client treatment and ensure payment for services you provide.

The strategies and skills you will learn in this book will work regardless of changes in insurance policies, the economy, or other unforeseen circumstances, enabling you to survive and thrive in practice. I experienced this directly soon after beginning my own practice in 1990. I had no idea then that the insurance industry was poised for a drastic overhaul. The next several years became a whirlwind of managed care takeovers, fee reductions, micromanagement, and bankruptcies. These and many other unexpected changes threatened my practice over the years, but I prevailed by using many of the strategies that I now offer here. Whether you desire a full- or part-time practice, they will also help you to thrive, even when the most unexpected occurs.

Acknowledgments

I would like to thank my colleagues, family, friends, and many others who assisted me in numerous ways to help create this book. I appreciate your helpful feedback on early drafts, your continual support and encouragement, and your belief in the value of this project. Thanks to all the mental health clinicians who so graciously shared their time and private practice experiences with me. With their invaluable help, readers can open the normally closed doors of private practice and learn from real-life challenges and triumphs. (To preserve confidentiality, I've changed practitioner and client names as well as identifying information within the chapters.) A special thanks to my editor, Deborah Malmud, at W. W. Norton & Company; I appreciate your expert feedback, direction, and professionalism which have remained constant from the very first day.

The following individuals have been instrumental to the success of this book:

Randee Allen, B.A.	Vivien Harvey, M.F.T.
Fred Alpern, Ph.D.	Laura Hawkins, B.A.
Karol Bailey, Ph.D.	Faye & Dennis Hunt
Diane Burch, C.P.A.	Teri Key, Ph.D.
Stephanie Calcagno, M.F.T.	Barrie Lamonte, L.C.S.W.
Andrew Chapman	Cynthia LaMotte, Ph.D.
Lorna Christensen, L.C.S.W.	Steven LaMotte, Ph.D.

Robert Cialidini, Ph.D.   Michael Lennie, Esq.

Barbara Cox, Ph.D.   Steven Meineke, M.F.T.

Matthew Duggan, Ph.D.   Doug Nies, Ph.D.

Rosalie Easton, Ph.D.   Margo Parker, Ph.D.

Michelle Felix, Ph.D.   Andrea Rosenbaum-Vogel, M.Ed.

Robert Goodman, Ph.D.   Lee Silber

                                       Katherine Taylor, L.C.S.W.

Essentials of Private Practice

PART I
Lowering Overhead Expenses

CHAPTER ONE

Arranging Your Practice Right from the Start

If you are thinking about starting a private practice or changing the way you already practice, the independence and flexibility of being your own boss has undeniable appeal. You don't have to follow someone else's schedule or job requirements, you get to call the shots and create your own practice. If you want to be a specialist, no problem—you can focus on your areas of interest and expertise. If you only want to work certain days, you decide. Anytime you change your mind, you can adjust your practice accordingly. In a world dominated by salaried employees working 40 to 60 hours a week, the option of professional self-employment is an enticing break from the norm.

However, you may have also heard frightening stories of others who were forced to shut down their practices when financially strapped. You may have been cautioned about being a private practitioner in this uncertain economic climate, with lower-paying managed care the dominant insurance, expenses on the rise, and a crowded field of many established clinicians.

There is no doubt that these factors make starting and maintaining a self-employed practice more challenging now than ever before. Many years ago therapists could set up shop with little thought to financial management; these days attending to your bottom line can be crucial to your success. Consider my colleague, Paula, who started her practice before managed care was established. She did not pay much attention to expenses before going solo, as high-paying indemnity insurance was prevalent at the time and she didn't need to see many clients each week in order to cover costs and earn a profit. Sure enough, with a little marketing, reimbursements from her small clientele quickly exceeded expenses and her practice grew.

Over time she upgraded to a very expensive office suite, filled it with fine leather and antique furnishings, and hired staff to take care of everything. However, when most of Paula's insured clients were switched from indemnity to lower-paid managed care coverage, she was forced to realize that she could no longer earn a living practicing the same way. She was working constantly to cover expenses, hoping each month to stay out of debt, and continually worrying about the bills. At times she even considered abandoning her financially strapped business. Fortunately, she was able to completely overhaul her practice, moving to a much smaller and affordable office, letting go of her staff, and choosing inexpensive furnishings to fit her new place. Paula is now doing well again, and can directly attest to the value of careful financial management.

This story illustrates the all-too-real monetary pitfalls that you can encounter in independent practice today. According to information reported in the April 2003 issue of *Psychotherapy Finances*, as many as 75 percent of practitioners do not have a business plan. You can avoid joining this majority of those who are vulnerable to financial hardships by following the steps described in the following pages. You will gain the advantage of setting up and maintaining your practice in the most cost-effective way, through careful budgeting and wise selection of the best arrangement for you. By considering the various options in working alone or with others and comparing the costs and benefits of each choice, you can reduce overhead expenses, lower stress, and maximize your take-home pay at the same time. Whether you plan to work part- or full-time, market a little or a lot, you will *always earn more by saving more*.

Secure an Income Base

If you are just starting or returning to a practice and do not have other financial support, it is best to have a steady job with guaranteed payment (e.g., salaried employment) to cover expenses before venturing out on your own. This approach protects you financially and helps to lower anxiety, preventing you from making stressful and costly mistakes out of fear. For instance, a newly licensed therapist I know rushed into a long-term office rental commitment before checking whether it matched her needs. She did not have a primary base of income and reacted out of financial fear and urgency to see clients and earn some money. She soon realized that the office was not very accessible or well maintained, and at night the area was not well lit or safe. Instead of quickly earning income, she struggled to build her clientele and was stuck in a year-long lease. If she had acquired a steady source of funds *before* starting out, she could have taken her time to choose the best office for her practice and avoided these hardships.

Most people secure an income base by working in a full- or part-time job and then taking a step into self-employment. For example, one clinician I know started by seeing clients in the evenings after his day job in the rehabilitation medicine department of a hospital. Another began by taking night appointments after working days at a university counseling center. I, too, kept a steady job in the beginning, transitioning from full- to part-time hours at the VA before seeing clients.

Estimate Basic Expenses

Once you have an income base, one of the best things you can do to ensure the fiscal health of your business is to estimate your practice expenses. You need a clear idea of start-up and monthly costs. You can then choose the arrangement you can afford, protecting yourself financially as you get started. Once you are established, by periodically reviewing your expenses compared to income, you will be able to spot money problems right away, allowing you to make whatever adjustments you need to to maintain profitability. Each time you lower costs, your earnings automatically rise, and the less you'll have to market or increase your client load to earn a profit.

If this is your first time practicing independently, congratulations! You have worked many years and very hard to reach the point of becoming your own boss. If you are re-entering practice, many aspects such as insurance plans, rates, office rental prices, and client/therapist ratios may have markedly changed in your absence. Although you do have extra costs when working for yourself, the good news is that now you can deduct a variety of business expenses that you could not as an employee. These deductions lower your net income and, in turn, reduce your taxes so you can keep more of what you earn.

Issue	Recommendation
Setting up and maintaining your practice in the most cost-effective way.	1) To protect yourself financially, secure an income base before entering private practice (pp. 1–3). 2) To help choose an affordable practice arrangement, estimate your practice expenses (pp. 2–3). 3) To create an efficient and profitable practice, periodically review and lower your expenses. (pp. 2–3).

Review Existing Expenses

The following are some items you may have already been paying for before entering private practice; if so, they will not add to your outlay in the beginning until your usage of them increases. In the options I describe shortly, you will see how starting out small can help minimize costs such as these until your income can support additional expenditure. Plus, entering private practice allows you to deduct these expenses in part or in full, provided they are professional costs incurred to generate earnings as a self-employed practitioner. To help in this process, it is also important to consult a licensed tax professional about any and all business related deductions.

- Books
- Classes/Seminars
- Dues/Subscriptions
- Supervision/consultation
- Internet
- Business Calls
- Postage
- Supplies
- Auto
- Meals/Entertainment
- Parking
- Travel

To estimate your costs in these areas, record the average amount you pay for each item per month. I've included a worksheet in Appendix A to assist you with this process. For expenses you pay quarterly, yearly, or at irregular intervals, convert them to monthly averages to allow for easy addition and comparison of costs. If you plan to add to or increase usage of any of these items after you become self-employed, you can do similar estimates based on projected monthly usage. For example, for Internet service, you can call companies to compare their typical monthly fees. For now, keep your business calls and supplies estimates to what you're currently paying to obtain baseline averages for these items. This will allow you to determine the basic expenses needed for the least expensive option of joining a group, where the extra costs for these items are typically covered. Later, you can add extra funds needed for solo and expense-sharing arrangements. As you become more familiar with this process, you will be able to quickly update estimates throughout your practice life. You can then compare expenses to income as your practice changes, allowing you to adjust items as necessary to maintain financial success.

Necessary Expenses

Regardless of the private practice arrangement you choose, you will also need to budget for these necessary items:

Item	Usually Paid
Professional License	Every Two Years
Business License	Yearly
Malpractice Insurance	Yearly or Quarterly
Continuing Education	Whenever Earning Hourly Credits for Relicensure

If you don't already have these expenses, you can call or search the Internet to estimate their costs. Your state licensing board and city office will have established amounts for license fees, and you can survey two or three malpractice insurance companies and average their quotes. To calculate continuing education costs, average hourly rates from two or three different workshops and multiply this by the number of hours required for relicensure.

After obtaining costs for each item, convert them to yearly and then monthly amounts to easily add and compare them with other costs. Follow a similar process for the list of recommended expenses described next, obtaining monthly average expenses for each one.

Recommended Expenses

Items recommended to fund any practice situation are:

Item	Usually Paid
Medical Insurance	Monthly
Disability Insurance	Quarterly or Monthly
Life Insurance	Quarterly or Monthly (if you have dependents)
Accounting Services	Quarterly or Yearly

Although these insurances are not required, when you switch from working for someone else to being your own boss, you no longer have the automatically paid benefits of insurance, sick and vacation days, and others to do your job when you are gone. If you are not covered by these insurances, a minor illness could pitch your practice into a financial danger zone, and a major emergency or chronic disease could shut your business down. According to information distributed by the American Psychological Association Insurance Trust in 2005, the risk of disability is greater than death at every age from 25 to 65. If you are 30, you have a 50 percent chance of becoming disabled for more than three months before age 65.

Imagine the stress of being laid up at home, losing income from clients you can't see, plus having to pay all medical bills. This happened to one of my colleagues, who had been practicing for five years when she began to suffer from multiple chronic illnesses that periodically required hospitalization for treatment. Fortunately, she had prepared for this hardship in advance by securing medical and disability insurance. When she became too ill to work, she was able to use her insurance benefits and avoid major financial stress, allowing her to stay in practice during her disability, treatment, and recovery.

Lowering Insurance Costs

You, too, can protect yourself and your practice from such a disaster by securing these policies right away. If you are unfortunate enough to become disabled and are incapable of performing the duties of your occupation, medical insurance will help cover medical expenses and disability insurance will replace a majority of your lost earnings. If you do not have any dependents, you may be able to skip life insurance, which would pay a certain amount upon your death, but the other two are crucial.

One way you can lower insurance costs is to obtain coverage from professional organizations, as they often provide lower group rates as well as discounts for multiple policies as a benefit of membership. For instance, you can get disability and malpractice insurance from the AAMFT, ACA, APA, and NASW and receive a good discount on these plans as a member. I found this out the hard way. After paying big fees to a large, well-known company for disability insurance for years, I compared costs with my national association's plan and realized I was paying about *three times* as much for the same coverage. With some checking, you may also be able to save a lot through these group plans, with the only caveat that you must remain a member of the group to keep your policies active.

Accounting Services

Although paying for an accountant does add an extra expense, once you become your own boss, even if you only work part-time, there are many new tax-related issues to address. Self-employment gets very complicated and laws change frequently. If you decide to do your own taxes, as one of my colleagues with a business background does, keep in mind that you will need to put in extra time and effort to research and adhere to rules to get the most from your tax return. If this work is not appealing, an accountant can help you navigate the system to reap the most benefits financially, quickly covering the cost of services by maximizing your take-home pay.

Many of the fees mentioned on pages 4–5 can already be deducted, including those paid to an accountant. However, if you don't know this you can really lose a lot. My friend Dawn lost thousands of dollars her first year out because she did her own taxes and didn't know all the ways she could retain more income by taking these self-employed deductions. She was used to working as an employee in her previous jobs, simply receiving a paycheck after her employers took care of financial matters such as taxes and deductions. After becoming self-employed, her mindset of working for someone else remained and she didn't transition to taking charge of these business details. As a result, she did not deduct business expenses she was entitled to and lost a lot of money she could have saved that year. For example, consider that if you pay $500 monthly for rent, you could deduct $6,000 a year for this expense alone.

One more expense you incur when working for yourself is self-employment tax, in which you pay a certain amount, let's say 7.65 percent, as an employer plus 7.65 percent as an employee. This is in addition to the income tax you pay on earnings, so it's even more crucial when self-employed to take all the deductions you can to offset this cost. An accountant can be your best ally to help you do this. This is the one outside service I have always paid for. My CPA, Diane, saves me much time and grief and more than pays for herself by maximizing my income. She also helps with quarterly tax payments, another new responsibility you will have when you are self-employed. I send her information every few months and receive an updated estimate of taxes due each quarter. By making accurate payments throughout the year, you can more easily monitor and adjust your budget to stay consistently in the black. You also prevent unpleasant end-of-the-year tax penalties for underpayment.

CHOOSING AN ACCOUNTANT. If you decide to use an accountant's services, it is very helpful to select someone experienced in providing services to private practitioners, and who ideally already has therapist clients. You can ask for such recommendations from fellow clinicians or from your local, regional, or national associations. If you don't have a personal referral, or even if you do, you can call prospective accountants and interview them to select one who works with clinicians. Start with the following questions: "Have you worked with therapists in self-employed private practice? Do you have any current clients who are self-employed clinicians? Could I contact one or more of these therapists as references for your services?"

By calling two or more accountants and asking for their customary fees, you can determine current market rates and keep this expense reasonable by avoiding someone who charges much more than the others. During your conversation you can also get a sense of who would be most compatible in meeting your needs and maintaining a good working alliance. Never underestimate your interpersonal acumen as a trained clinician to guide you. If any nagging feelings surface, pay attention to them, they may be your best aid in finding the right accountant for the long term.

Once you obtain references, call them as well to ask about their experiences. You might ask them: "Were you satisfied in general with your accountant's services? Did he/she spend adequate time answering questions and thoroughly reviewing your individual needs as a self-employed

Issue	Recommendation
Obtaining insurances and accounting services for your private practice.	1) To financially protect yourself and your loved ones in case of an unexpected health crisis, secure medical, disability, and life insurance (pp. 5–6). 2) To keep these insurance costs low, compare rates and purchase them from your professional organizations (pp. 6–7). 3) To maximize your take-home pay, hire an accountant to help with self-employed tax issues (pp. 7–8). 4) To choose an accountant, interview two or more to find one who is reasonably priced and most compatible in meeting your needs (pp. 7–9).

clinician? Did you feel you received the most deductions and suggestions for maximizing your net income? Were services performed in a timely manner and reasonably priced?"

Totaling Basic Expenses

Once you obtain estimates for these basic expenses—the existing, necessary, and recommended expenses detailed earlier (see pp. 4–5)—add them together on the worksheet in Appendix A. The total will be the bottom line amount you will need to pay monthly as a self-employed practitioner. Additional costs of setting up your own office, such as rent and equipment, are purposely not included in this total. This allows you to first check whether you have enough for the least expensive option of joining a group, described next, where additional office overhead would already be covered. If you have more than enough available funds, you may be able to afford the most expensive option of setting up your own office. However, if not, you still have another mid-priced option of sharing expenses with others, where you would be responsible for *some* additional costs such as rent and billing.

As you continue reading and deciding what practice choice you prefer, by estimating the costs required, you can evaluate your ability to pay for that choice and develop a plan to acquire what you need before starting out. For example, you may have just enough to join a group practice even though you'd really like to have your own office someday. By estimating costs and saving ahead, you could start in a group, transition to subletting office space, and later set up your own office once you can afford the extra outlay required. By taking this approach, you avoid the disaster of overextending yourself financially and panicking when there is no money for bills that come due.

Unfortunately, this is exactly what happened to my colleague's friend, who did not estimate basic costs or additional office fees before deciding on the most expensive option of setting up his own practice. He rented a high-priced office and bought the best furnishings and equipment without considering whether he could afford them with current funds. He assumed he would quickly be seeing enough clients to more than cover these bills. When his client load did not build as expected, he was stuck trying to keep up with expenses and after seven months closed down his practice. If he had estimated costs ahead of time, he could have prevented this disaster and chosen a more affordable arrangement matched to his existing resources, where he could stay as long as needed to build a clientele. Knowing your expenses, especially in the beginning, you can protect yourself by making sure you have enough discretionary money to pay for the practice arrangement you want before starting out on your own.

Joining a Group

If your cost analysis reveals that you can afford basic expenses but no more, your least expensive self-employed option is to join an existing group that pays for additional overhead costs. In this arrangement, you typically become an independent contractor, signing an agreement to give a certain percentage of your total earnings to the group in exchange for these benefits. If at first you earn nothing, you pay nothing; however, the means are available to build your clientele. Although part of the group, this contract establishes you as self-employed versus an employee, with the advantage that now you can write off many of your basic expenses as business deductions.

If you'd eventually like to have your own practice, a group can provide a useful stepping-stone toward this goal. This is how I got started in private practice. After downshifting to part-time hours at the VA, I joined a group because it was inexpensive and less intimidating at the time compared to going solo. I liked the idea of gaining clinical and business experience in a group while building more confidence and income to go out on my own. Since it was a large group with offices in many locations, I was able to work in two different cities and decide which one I preferred before putting down roots in a solo arrangement.

Maybe your goals are different and you don't care to go out on your own someday. Perhaps you have extra funds but you don't want to spend them on a more costly individual practice. You may not want all the responsibility of setting up and managing a business, and the idea of working in a group, in which someone else assumes more financial risk, is more appealing. Perhaps there are other endeavors you'd like to pursue, but you'd still like to be your own boss part-time within a group, where there are other colleagues around for professional or social contact.

Whatever your reason for joining a group, a major benefit is that you can receive everything you need right away to see clients, at no extra expense to you. Usually you're provided office space, secretarial and billing services, client referrals, phone/pager usage, supplies, stationery, etc. If you do testing or use specialized therapy supplies, the group may already have assessment and treatment materials you can use. If not, you could negotiate to cover their cost, saving you from this added expense. You could also request payment for the basic practice expenses already listed, but most groups do not cover individual professional costs, such as license fees and malpractice/disability insurance premiums.

Some people choose the group option by default, if they are already working in a group as an employed intern or psychological assistant and then negotiate to change to a self-employed position after licensure. You may get lucky like my internship colleague, Anita, who was asked after becoming licensed to stay on with the group she had worked for, continuing in her new independent status with a full client load she had built over the previous two years. However, you are much more likely to have to initiate this request yourself. I'd recommend approaching the leader early on after you start working for a group and before you become licensed. By specifically asking for what you want, you will increase your chances of staying with the group after licensure.

You can also do this if you are working elsewhere and wish to join a group. A clinician I know named David walked to every mental health practice in the office building near his full-time agency job, picking up business cards from their offices and making cold calls. Although only one called him back, that was all he needed, and soon thereafter he was offered a position in the group. By doing your own research and assertively stepping out, you, too, can get what you want. If you don't initiate, no one will know you are there or what you are looking for.

Issue	Recommendation
Weighing the practice option of joining a group (as an independent contractor).	1) After completing your basic expense estimate, check whether you can afford this monthly total. If so, consider joining a group, where they would cover additional overhead costs (pp. 9–11). 2) To help in your decision, assess whether your career goals and personal preferences are compatible with this group arrangement (pp. 9–11).

Selecting a Group

If you decide to join a group, the following are some items to watch out for before committing and signing an agreement. Although you may not run into any problems, these issues are helpful to consider so you can protect yourself financially, ethically, and legally.

Background Check

When looking for a group, you can find out who is in your area and what their reputation is by asking anyone who might know such as friends, colleagues, supervisors and co-workers. You can also search professional publications, the yellow pages, the Internet, or other directories for leads. My colleague, Jennifer, found a group by attending an annual professional association meeting and asking practitioners there for recommendations. It turned out that two group leaders were also at the meeting, and she was able to interview both during breaks, quickly deciding on which group to pursue further.

After identifying a potential group, another way to check out the leaders and/or members is by verifying their credentials through state licensing boards, a strategy that is especially helpful if no one knows these clinicians. After obtaining their license type and name, you can call or log onto the appropriate state website and typically receive their current license status and previous practice history, including any complaints filed. If you know additional details such as their full name and city of practice, your search may be even faster. If you find any questionable information, you could either address it directly or simply move on to another group. The Internet search option was not available when I was deciding on a group. Now, with a few keystrokes, you can access much information through licensing and other professional websites at your convenience.

PAYMENT. Even after a thorough background check, undetected problems with groups can slip through. Consider what happened to my friend Valerie, who, soon after becoming licensed, agreed to join a group that provided services to a hospital. They offered to bill the hospital for her work and pay her a reasonable percentage of earnings, as soon as compensation was first received from the hospital. Valerie provided group and individual therapy, putting in many hours weekly, but received nothing in return. Upon inquiry, she was told that since the group hadn't been paid, there was no money to give her and she would need to wait.

The weeks stretched into months, and each time she asked, she was told the same thing. She ended up working more than a year until the group leaders suddenly left the country and were nowhere to be found. Other therapists involved with this group were stuck in a similar situation, with months of unpaid work, and many of them pursued legal actions against the leaders. Although this happened over fifteen years ago, the legal and financial aftermath is still dragging on. Fortunately Valerie was able to cut her losses and move on, eventually relocating to another state and starting her own private practice, where she is doing well to this day.

Although this disaster may not happen to you, any number of less extreme payment problems could derail you financially and spike your stress level. To protect yourself before joining a group, you can talk with the leader to clarify your exact payment percentage. For example, my arrangement was 60/40; I kept 60 percent of earnings and gave 40 percent to the group. From interviews with others, this appears to be a common percentage agreement, with a general range between 70/30 and 50/50. In my case, a graduated commission scale offered 63 percent to me if I grossed a certain amount monthly, and 66 percent if I earned even more, etc.

You can also protect yourself by ensuring a written contract is offered. In Valerie's situation, since her agreement was verbal, she was left with little recourse to recoup her unpaid services. Even if a small issue arises for you, it will be much easier to hold someone accountable when you have the original agreement in writing. Once you receive the contract, it is in your best interest to read it carefully before you sign. If you have any contract concerns or questions, consider obtaining legal advice. Professional organizations are a good referral resource to find attorneys familiar with mental health contracts, and if you are a member, you may get limited service at no cost or at a significant discount. You can also contact malpractice insurance companies for attorney referrals; if you already have a policy or plan to purchase one, you may be entitled to a no-cost consultation with one of their in-house attorneys. Keep in mind that you can negotiate anything you don't like in the contract beforehand, including your percentage rate. When you already have a source of income, it's easier to stay strong in what you want, taking as much time as you need to find the right group.

Another important issue to address is how soon you will be paid after rendering services; this should be ideally thirty and no longer than sixty days. For added protection, make sure this is specified in the contract, along with your agreed upon payment rate and other negotiated details.

You now know what Valerie didn't—you should never have to wait months to receive payment unless you've already agreed to it in writing.

BILLING. Another way to prevent payment problems is to find out ahead of time who will be billing for your services, asking to personally meet him/her to explain how your pay is calculated and reported. During your meeting, request a contact number you can call whenever you have questions. Once you start working, you can compare your record of services to billing reports and payments you should be getting every month. If you don't receive anything or there are discrepancies, you can call your billing contact right away to find out why. Sometimes it may be a simple computer or accounting error, and can be fixed right away. However, if the same error occurs a second or third month, there may be a bigger problem. You can either take the issue to a higher power or leave the group, before being stuck like Valerie with months of work and no income.

If you are already familiar with billing practices, you may consider negotiating to do your own, avoiding the work of double-checking payments. If so, keep in mind that it will take more time, effort, and expense to do this and as a compensation, it is in your best interest to discuss lowering the earnings percentage you give to the group. However, in most cases, and especially if you are just getting started, you will probably opt for the group to take care of the billing. This is why watching your payment is so important. No one cares about your money quite like you do and these steps will help you get paid exactly what you have earned.

Referrals

Another important area to address before selecting a group is referrals. Be sure to clarify with the leader how and when you will be getting new clients, adding this to your contract as well. Although the assumption is usually that as a group member you will receive referrals, when this is made explicit you are in a much better position to hold the group accountable if this does not happen. Once you join, immediately monitor your referrals and compare them to your agreement, addressing any discrepancies right away.

This strategy can help you avoid what happened to Linda, a newly-licensed therapist who expected new clients right away after joining a group. Her first referral did not come until three months later, after she had gone through most of her personal savings and was stressed to her limit. She ended up leaving the group for an agency job, but plans to get

Issue	Recommendation
Protecting yourself legally, ethically, and financially before committing to a group.	1) To locate group options, ask professionals you know and search publications, the Internet, and other directories for leads (p. 12). 2) To screen groups for ethical and legal problems, verify members' credentials and practice history, addressing questionable information or moving on to consider another group (pp. 12–13). 3) To ensure accurate and timely payment, clarify in your contract your exact payment percentage and timeframe to be paid (pp. 12–14). 4) To protect yourself legally before joining a group, consult an attorney to review contract details and receive specific legal advice (p. 13). 5) To prevent payment delays, personally meet the billing specialist before joining a group, so later you can address any payment discrepancies with him/her right away (p. 14).

back into private practice once her finances are secure, where you can be sure she will be clarifying referrals up front and in writing, closely watching and addressing problems right away.

Policies and Procedures

You can also prevent many problems by clarifying how your clients are scheduled, the hours you will work, and what office space you can use. When Linda investigated her lack of referrals, she learned that she had not been added to the computer-scheduling database, a crucial step in being eligible for new client referrals. By finding out exactly how staff assigns clients, you can take whatever steps are needed to ensure you get referrals as soon as possible. Clarifying the screening process of referrals will also help you to make sure your referrals match your areas of competence and comfort. My colleague Jennifer discovered soon after joining a group that she was routinely assigned to see clients on Saturdays. She had assumed that she would be working weekday evenings, but she hadn't clarified these hours or added them to the written contract before she started working in the group. If Jennifer had addressed her hours before committing to the group, she could have negotiated to obtain the schedule she wanted or rearranged other commitments to free her Saturdays to see clients.

Especially in large groups with limited office space, by clearly identifying what space you can use and when, you can avoid the stressful experience of coming to the office and finding someone else using your room. Another clinician named Tim came to what he assumed was his office one day to find all of his personal things taken from his desk drawer, including his diplomas and an expensive clock. Luckily he found them in another office and was told that since there was limited space, he should put all his things in a box and carry them from office to office, depending on which one was available. Although you may not always be able to avoid problems like this, by addressing these and other issues ahead of time, you increase the chances of identifying and solving potential problems before they surface, or simply moving on to another group.

Staff

Another important issue to check out is the office staff, especially how they deal with clients and you. Whatever group you affiliate yourself with will reflect on you, so you want to be sure to avoid working with someone who projects an unprofessional manner, especially in our field of therapeutic work. My friend Dawn worked in a group with a very stern office manager. Although she was very good at collecting fees, clients became noticeably upset after interacting with her. Dawn found she was spending more and more time helping people work through their reactions to this manager, with less time focused on the real reasons they came to therapy.

After a while, this office manager was replaced by someone completely different. Instead of a severe demeanor, she was overly friendly with clients waiting for their appointments, learning about their personal lives, therapy issues, and even giving advice. Dawn soon noticed her clients engaging in therapy much differently, and often at cross-purposes to identified therapy goals and steps. It turns out that neither of these extreme styles was helpful to clients or the therapy process. By observing staff ahead of time you can see if they are harsh, too involved, or otherwise unprofessional, and if so address the problems or move on.

You can also check to see whether staff completes tasks in a timely manner and exactly what paperwork they give to clients. Anything disseminated by the group will reflect on you, so it's important to make sure it meets ethical, legal, and professional guidelines.

Leaving a Group

One helpful point to add to your group contract before signing is the option to resign by giving thirty days written notice. Then, if you discover any of these problems after joining, you can easily get out by simply giving notice. Another item to take out of your contract is any clause preventing you from continuing to see existing clients after leaving the group. Then, if you do decide to resign, your clients will have the option to continue services with you wherever you go. These issues may become especially important if your goal is to move on to your own or a different practice at some point. By attending to them in advance, you can facilitate a smooth transition when you're ready.

Issue	Recommendation
Selecting a well-run group that meets your clients' needs as well as your own.	1) To ensure referrals, clarify in advance how and when you will be getting new clients (pp. 15–16). 2) To prevent problems in the office, clarify your work hours, how your clients are scheduled, and what office space you will use (pp. 14–15). 3) To ensure quality staff, observe how they relate to clients; address problems before joining the group or move on to consider another one (p. 16). 4) To facilitate leaving a group, add to your contract the option to quickly resign; remove any clause preventing you from continuing to treat your clients after you leave (p. 17).

Going Solo

After reading about the group option, you may be thinking, "Well, I'd like to eventually have an individual practice, but for now I'll start in a group and work my way toward this goal." Maybe you're not sure how long it will take to afford going out on your own. Or you might want more clinical experience or group camaraderie before going solo. Although you may think going solo is far off, you could be surprised by how quickly you can afford this option once you estimate the extra expenses required and save the investment you need. Six months after joining a group, I did this and found out that I could afford to leave right away if I wanted. If I hadn't done these calculations, I may have stayed much longer without realizing I had another option that I found more attractive.

Maybe instead you're saying to yourself, "I don't care to join a group, but I would like to go out on my own." You may desire the freedom and independence that comes with having your own office and making all the decisions. If you can easily afford basic expenses required in joining a group, you may be in a good position to consider setting up your own practice. A major advantage to this is complete control over everything; however, the downside is that you will need to pay for additional office expenses and do everything yourself.

Estimating Expenses

Whether or not you have a clearly defined practice goal, by calculating extra expenses needed to go solo, you can determine if and when this is the right choice for you. The following list covers additional start-up and ongoing expenses you will need to pay if you set up your own office. By estimating these and adding them to your previously determined basic expenses, you can determine the total you will need for an independent practice (see Appendix B).

Additional Start-Up Expenses	Examples
Security Deposit	First and last month's rent
Furnishings	Furniture, pictures, plants, magazine subscriptions
Equipment	Fax, copier, computer, printer
Communications systems	Phones and set-up fees, pager, answering service/machine
Billing (option 1, billing software)	Computer software
Testing and therapy tools	WAIS-R, play therapy toys
Additional Ongoing Expenses	**Examples**
Rent	Monthly rent
Office overhead insurance	Quarterly or yearly payments
Business owner's insurance	Quarterly or yearly payments
Equipment supplies/repairs	Paper, disks, computer repair
Communications fees	Monthly calling plans, voicemail fees
Billing (option 2, billing service)	Monthly services
Other supplies	Business cards, stationery, claim forms
Advertising	Yellow pages, Internet, publications

Ways to Keep Expenses Low

As you go through these lists, keep in mind that many items, such as office furnishings and equipment, you will only need to purchase once to get started. You retain control over acquiring new items for your office once it's set up; by spending conservatively you can easily keep these expenses low.

You can also keep costs down by looking for less expensive but still professionally appropriate items, surveying two or more places for prices and calculating an average estimate for each one. Remember Paula, whose story I described in the beginning? She estimated her furniture expense this way, averaging prices in some large, well-known stores and eventually choosing the most reasonable offer. These days you can compare costs many ways, by reading paper ads, making phone calls, searching the Internet, and directly visiting retailers. Often high-volume stores will have the best prices and special deals. Be sure to keep your detective work together in a safe place so when you're ready to buy, you can use it to guide your purchases.

You can also compare office rents in a similar way, by searching professional publications and websites for ads, asking colleagues for leads, and driving to areas in which you'd like to practice to find rental signs. You will read more about this in Chapter 2, which guides you in selecting a reasonably priced office that matches your needs.

Office Equipment

Chances are, you probably have some items listed on page 18 already, such as a computer, printer, fax, or cellular phone. If so, you will save by avoiding these start-up costs; plus now you can start deducting related supplies and usage fees (e.g., cartridges, calling plan). A suitable computer may be your biggest expense. You can make this easier by budgeting and saving for this purchase well ahead of time. I keep this expense low by never buying the newest or fastest model. Instead, I choose a computer powerful enough for the applications I use, but without the extra features I don't need.

As technology advances, equipment costs often go down. For example, these days you can get a combination fax/copier/printer for a very reasonable price. Or if you want to buy them separately, fax and printers are more easily affordable than they were years ago. Depending on your usage needs, an office copy machine may be more expensive. I cut this cost in half by buying a display model. It appeared in good condition and the sales agent confirmed it had been sitting out a short time with limited usage. Just in case of a needed repair, it did come with a warranty. I've had it four years now and still use it with no problems. By looking for these kinds of discounts, you can save a lot in your purchases.

Note that installation and calling plan fees are usually more expensive for a business versus personal telephone line, so it's especially helpful to get estimates ahead of time to aid in your communications set-up. Consider my office neighbor Melanie's experience: she ordered phone lines for her new office, assuming they would cost the same as her home line. After four business lines were already installed, she was stunned upon opening her much larger-than-expected bill. If she had known these higher costs beforehand, she would have limited her order to one or two lines instead of the four she thought were well within her budget. You can avoid an unexpected bill by calling ahead and comparing prices, choosing only what you need and can afford at the time.

Billing and Supplies

You also have choices in handling billing. To help you decide, you can compare prices of billing software (option 1) versus outside billing services (option 2). You can even handwrite bills and avoid this expense altogether, especially in the beginning. This is what I did at first, using a manual recording system for appointments, fees, and writing out claims to insurance. However, these days you can get reasonably priced billing software that is also user-friendly. You may be surprised how easy it can be to do it yourself versus paying someone else, saving you a lot in the long run. You will read more about this recommended option in Chapter 6.

Additional supplies such as business cards and stationary don't have to be fancy; you can buy good quality at reasonable prices from office service and supply stores. I just bought 1,000 business cards with raised-letter printing at my neighborhood store for less than the price of a large pizza. Of course, you can always print out stationary and business cards yourself, but be careful, especially with business cards, as they can easily look unprofessional if they have rough edges, smudge easily, or are too flimsy.

Advertising

You can also keep advertising expenses to a minimum, based on your needs and budget. Keep in mind that there are ways to market your services at no extra cost, such as member listings in professional directories and association websites. Plus, if you join insurance panels, you will likely get free advertising on their provider websites and directories. How much additional exposure you want can vary; you can always start small to keep expenses low and adjust as desired.

Issue	Recommendation
Considering a solo practice option.	1) To determine whether you can afford a solo practice, do a second expense estimate, factoring in career goals and personal preferences in your decision (pp. 17–18). 2) In looking for less expensive quality items, obtain two or more price estimates and put them in a safe place for easy access when you're ready to buy (p. 19). 3) Budget for large purchases in advance, and reduce expenditures by buying only what you need (p. 21). 4) Obtain office overhead and business owner's insurance, which will cover practice expenses if you become disabled and office contents you could lose in a disaster (pp. 19–21).

Additional Insurance

Two more recommended expenses when renting your own office are office overhead and business owner's insurance. Like the other insurances mentioned, you can obtain these through your professional organizations. Office overhead insurance protects you if you become disabled, paying your ongoing office expenses until you can get back to work. Remember my colleague, who suffered from many chronic illness and repeated hospitalizations? Fortunately, she was also covered by this insurance and was able to maintain her office until she could return to work. As I watched this happen to her, a relatively young woman, I learned a valuable personal lesson. If I hadn't witnessed these hardships afflict my colleague, I may not have recognized the need for such protection for myself. Business owner's insurance will protect what's inside your office in the event of a fire, burglary, or other disaster causing comprehensive damage to your office. You will be reimbursed for any insured losses including expensive items like furniture, paintings, computer, and other business machines. These funds will allow you to replace what you need in your office and continue your business without extra financial strain.

Expense Sharing

When reviewing these additional costs, perhaps you're not quite financially ready or willing to go entirely on your own yet. Maybe your plan is to join a group and transition to individual practice, but your estimate reveals the start-up solo expenses are higher than you expected. You may not know just when you'll be able to pay for everything needed to go on your own. Or maybe you have no plans to join a group, but you don't want to be completely on your own either. If you are new to practice, you may not know yet where you will settle for the long term, and you'd rather not invest a lot or be stuck with a long rental commitment in one place.

Perhaps you have no desire to build a full-time practice, but you would like a small part-time one. You could have a full-time job you want to keep, such as teaching or research, but you'd like to see a few clients to keep your clinical skills sharp and earn extra income. Maybe you're a parent and want more time at home with your children, but you still want an active professional practice and enough income to pay certain expenses. Perhaps you want to follow other pursuits like painting or travel, but you'd still like to see some clients and earn a certain level of income.

Whatever your unique situation, an affordable way to solve these kinds of dilemmas and still practice independently is to share expenses with others. For example, you could sublet office space from a fellow clinician who is already established. This is much less expensive than setting up your own office, because you can minimize many start-up and ongoing costs. When expenses are lower, your take-home pay will increase without the need to build a big practice. In fact, by keeping your client load and income at a moderate level, you can stay in a lower tax bracket and limit this money drain, too.

Finding an Affordable Arrangement

Your best resources to find these opportunities are to ask colleagues and search publications and websites. For example, local professional associations frequently have monthly newsletters and websites listing available expense-sharing practice options. I found my first office to sublet right under my nose, in the office building where I worked as a group member. In talking with therapists in a neighboring suite, I discovered that they had an office I could rent part-time for a very affordable monthly fee. After estimating subletting costs, I compared the total to what I was paying the group at the time. To my surprise, I realized that not only could I afford to go on my own this way, but the take-home pay would be more than if I stayed with the group. By that time I had been with the group over six months, earning enough steady income from a small clientele to more than pay for the subletting expenses. With this knowledge, I quickly gave thirty-days notice and left the group to rent the space myself. By asking around and doing your own expense estimates, you can find affordable opportunities, perhaps in the places you least expect.

As you survey opportunities, by obtaining two or more options and comparing costs of each, you can ensure that they are within a reasonable range. To estimate expenses in an expense-sharing arrangement, go back to your solo expense worksheet in Appendix B and adjust or delete any items that will change. Then, recalculate totals to financially compare each choice. For instance, if one of your options involves renting a fully furnished office, you can delete the start-up furnishings expense. If you are considering arrangements of paying by the hour, day, or other part-time usage, you can greatly reduce your initial security deposit and ongoing monthly rent payments. My first rent was lowered when I paid for halftime usage; another clinician used it the rest of the time.

Reducing Expenses

You could also lower costs on equipment, communications systems, and/or supplies fees by negotiating to use systems that are already set up in an office. This could be arranged through the rental agreement or for a separate monthly fee. For example, another office neighbor, Susan, requested to use the copy and fax machines, telephone, and supplies while subletting her office. She suggested paying a fixed monthly amount for this usage, and her colleagues agreed to this arrangement. When I shared an office suite with two other therapists, we also lowered many of our costs by splitting them equally. In addition to the rent, we contributed to pay for common area furnishings (e.g., in waiting and conference rooms), equipment/repairs, phone service, kitchen and office supplies, and drinking water.

If you choose to share expenses but you'd still like your own office someday, you can prepare for this by monitoring your income, periodically updating your solo expense estimate, and then transitioning to your own office once you can afford the extra costs. Consider Susan's example: She started out subletting a furnished office by the hour, beginning with one evening after her agency day job. As her clientele grew and she could afford more, she added a second night and so on, until she expanded from an hourly to a half-time rental agreement. During this process, she transitioned to part-time hours at her day job, when her self-employed income was large enough to replace her salary loss. Eventually her practice grew; she expanded her rental agreement from half- to full-time, and left the agency. She furnished her space in her own style, paying in cash, and continues in full-time practice to this day, in the same office in which she started over twenty years ago.

If you are already working in your own office but would like to lower your costs, you can also sublet unused space to someone else. My colleague, Bill, did this by changing his schedule to see his entire clientele in two days. He moved all paperwork and non-client tasks home and rented his office to another clinician to use while he was gone. His children were small at the time and he did this primarily to spend more time at home with them. He soon realized that he liked the extra time and rental savings so much that he has continued this schedule ever since, even though his children are now adults living on their own.

There is really no limit to how creative you can be when you share expenses with others. It is to your advantage to take your time to review and implement these and other cost-saving options throughout your practice life. You will be rewarded with much lower overhead costs and higher take-home pay, even with a small clientele.

Issue	Recommendation
Considering an expense-sharing practice option.	1) To find expense-sharing opportunities, ask colleagues and search publications and/or websites (pp. 22–23). 2) For each option that you consider, go back to your solo expense estimate and reduce or delete any items that will change. Then recalculate totals to financially compare your choices (p. 23). 3) To lower expenses throughout your practice life, consider subletting space, dividing fees for commonly used items, and other cost-sharing strategies (pp. 23–24). 4) To transition to a solo office, periodically monitor your income, update your solo expense estimate, and move once you can afford the extra costs (pp. 23–24).

CHAPTER TWO

Choosing an Office That Fits Your Practice

In any practice option you are considering, an important decision you will make is choosing the office where you will work. By evaluating important factors such as location, safety, accessibility, specific features, and expenses ahead of time, you can select the best office to lower your stress, reduce costs, and maximize client satisfaction. Whether you are looking for your first office or relocating after many years, this one decision alone can bring you greater happiness at work, more clients, and higher take-home pay at the same time.

Remember Paula? She initially rented a very expensive office in an exclusive area of town. Everything about it was ideal for her except the cost. It was in a beautiful and very safe area, easily accessible by freeways and near her desired clientele. Since the office matched her practice needs and insurances were paying well at the time, she didn't think much about the rent and moved in. We already know what happened next; eventually she was forced to move to stay in practice. However, she found a way to stay in the same area at a much lower cost. With a little research, she found a much smaller, well-maintained office in an older nearby building. Her new location was within walking distance of her previous one and retained all the desirable features she wanted. Most importantly, it was one-fourth the rent! Paula's experience shows that you don't have to sacrifice the practice features that are most important to you to find an affordable office. With a little planning, you can find an office to fit your priorities and help you stay financially viable at the same time.

Location and Clientele

To help make your choice, two important questions to ask yourself are, "In what kind of neighborhood do I want to practice?" and "What type of clients do I want to work with?" Every area, spanning from the East to West Coast, whether urban or rural, has a unique identity and ambiance. Furthermore, communities can change abruptly when traveling from one to the next. If you've ever crossed a state, city, or county line and experienced a whole different world on the other side, you know what that's like. The same holds true for smaller neighborhoods whose character can change from block to block. In your search, look for an area where you would be comfortable and one that matches your style. You will be happier at work and more buffered from stress. Potential clients will also be influenced by your office location, from its closest cross streets to the surrounding city, county, and beyond. By identifying whom you want to work with, you can choose a location that also appeals to your clients in atmosphere, comfort, and convenience. With these factors in your favor, your referrals and earnings will automatically increase. You'll also save the time and cost of marketing and advertising efforts you would have to expend to draw people to a less-than-desirable location.

My colleague, Jim, went through a detailed decision-making process before choosing his full-time private practice office. At the time he was working in an inpatient substance abuse program at a medical hospital. His supervisor had just told him that the unit would be shut down in a few months and he was considering his options. Although he was offered another hospital position with a psychiatric unit, he decided that he really wanted to transition to full-time private practice. By that time he had been subletting an office for a while and had acquired a small but steady clientele. The location was satisfactory but didn't really match his style. He was laid back and casual, but his office sat in the middle of the city's bustling business district. Whenever he went to work, he tensed up, feeling like a fish out of water. He knew he wanted to be somewhere else within the city, but he wasn't exactly sure where. Although many of his outpatient clients were individuals and his inpatient job was exclusively adults, his real passion was working with families and children.

Keeping his preferences in mind, he set out on a drive to see what offices were available in different areas. Almost right away he saw a building with an office rental sign. It was near two elementary schools and surrounded by family homes, neighborhood restaurants, and other small businesses.

In the back was a basketball hoop and plenty of space for outside activities. A sidewalk in the front wound around to a nearby park. He intuitively knew this location was the right match for him, and after checking other places to be sure, he came back and rented the office. Although the rent was a little higher than his old one, he figured the atmosphere and potential referrals were worth the extra investment. He was much happier in the new location and his practice began to grow. Existing clients had no problem coming to the new office, as it was in the same city and just a ten-minute drive from the old one. New referrals started to come in from the nearby children and families he had deliberately relocated to see. When his inpatient unit shut down a few months later, he had enough steady income to leave the hospital and continue building his practice.

Although your situation may be different from Jim's, you can find your ideal office by answering the same two crucial questions I mentioned earlier: "In what kind of neighborhood do I want to practice?" and "What type of clients do I want to work with?" As he discovered, your answers are likely to converge. For example, perhaps you wish to work with patients coping with chronic pain or other health problems. You may be comfortable in an office near a hospital and physicians' offices, allowing easy access for patients with frequent medical visits and the opportunity for more referral possibilities within this community. Or you may prefer a clientele in corporate or other business positions, offering services such as career development and stress/time management. In this case, an office complex or high rise in a city's business district might appeal to your interests, offering busy executives convenient, quick, and private access to you. You may instead favor a clientele interested in alternative healing approaches. If so, an office near specialists such as acupuncturists, massage therapists, herbalists, and energy healers may reflect your preferred specialty and be conducive to desired referrals. There are many more possibilities for your location based on your preferences, and by taking the time to identify them you can match the best neighborhood to your desired clients and yourself at the same time.

Locate for the Long Term

Recall that when Jim moved, his ongoing clients could easily continue seeing him in his new office because it wasn't too far from the old one. Before you decide on your location, it's also helpful to ask yourself whether or not you plan to stay practicing in the same general area. By choosing an area where you envision staying for a long time, you can retain your clients and referral sources, and avoid having to network all over again. Even if you do move offices like Jim, as long as you do not move too far away, you can keep these practice foundations in place and preserve your income during the transition. Since I started in private practice, I have had three different office locations within a five-mile radius in the same city. Clients were able to easily follow me each time to my new office. Now many of my new referrals are people I've already seen in past years or friends and family they've referred to me. If I had moved much farther away, I know I'd be spending a lot more time and money marketing all over again—not something I really want to do.

Perceptual Boundaries

Another issue to factor into your decision of location is that potential clients often set their own boundaries of places they will and will not go. These perceptual limits can affect whether people seek you out for therapy. For example, my friend, Laura, practices in a city at the northern edge of a county. Although she's near the border of a neighboring county, and even though some of her clients live in cities that are closer or more convenient than those in her own county, she receives few new clients from there. People may feel more comfortable driving in areas they identify as their territory, such as their city and county. They may avoid places outside their boundaries, even if they are closer or the area is more freeway accessible. Many new clients find practitioners by searching their insurance directories, which usually group them by license type and city of practice. It's likely that clients automatically look for referrals within their city first, especially when they don't know the neighborhoods of offices in surrounding cities.

If many of your referrals come from an indirect method, locating within your desired city and county lines can help bring in the clients you would like to see. This issue may be lessened if you have many direct, personal referrals, but if you are starting out, you may not know yet just how your clients will find you. When your office is in the county and city where your desired clients live, you are optimally positioned for referrals regardless of the method by which they are received.

Locating in an Affluent Area

When making their choice, many therapists intentionally locate in an area primarily because it has affluent residents. These are typically desirable neighborhoods filled with professional, high-income people—a ready-made pool of potential clients. Sounds pretty good, right? Well, before you set your mind exclusively on this strategy, make sure to factor in your personal and client preferences mentioned earlier. Office rents in these areas can be high, so you want to make sure it's worth the expense to be there. Consider also that just like you, many other therapists are drawn to wealthy areas, creating increased competition for the same finite group of referrals. Before setting down roots in a potentially saturated location, you can save yourself unexpected grief by checking out how many clinicians may already be there. An easy way to find established therapists is to search the phone book or Internet directories (e.g., www.yellowpages.com).

My first private practice office was actually two, each in a different city provided through my group. Upon comparing yellow pages listings, I found similar numbers of therapists in both cities, even though one city had half the population of the other. Soon after working in each city, I noticed differences in overall client populations. Those in the less-populated city tended to be more affluent, married, and Caucasian. Clients in the more populated city were more middle-income and diverse in marital status and ethnicity. Although the latter clientele generally had lower-paying insurance and fewer self-pay referrals, I quickly realized I preferred working with them. I liked the greater diversity of issues and backgrounds and the chance to see more individuals versus couples or families. When I left the group practice I chose the larger city in which to develop my full-time practice based on my experiences and preferences. Since there were fewer therapists serving these residents, I also had an advantage in building a practice there—more potential clients and fewer local therapists. In my case it would have been a mistake to locate in the less-populated city even though there I would have had more affluent referrals. Expanding your decision beyond the wealth of a community to match your interests with your prospective clientele will allow you to enjoy a more successful practice in the long run. You will minimize burnout by doing the work you like, enhancing future referrals and creating a more stable income.

Balancing the Costs

If it turns out that your preferences are well suited to a wealthy area, but you still have concerns about rental prices, there are ways to locate there without going in the red. You could carefully shop around like Paula did, comparing rents of different offices in the area you want to be. From these options you could choose a less expensive one that retains the features that are most important to you.

If, like Jim, you really have your heart set on an office that costs more, you may decide it's worth the investment. Just as he did, you may find that your increased clientele over time more than covers the rental expense. You could also lower other costs to balance the added outlay. As described earlier, you could sublet, share expenses, comparison shop, and carefully buy only what you need and will use. In the following chapters you will read more about ways to lower other major expenses. By deciding what's most important to you, you can invest in your top priorities and make adjustments in other areas to balance things out.

Issue	Recommendation
Finding the right office location for you.	1) To increase your happiness and reduce stress at work, look for a neighborhood where you will be comfortable practicing and that matches your style (pp. 25–27). 2) To increase referrals of your desired clients, choose a location appealing to them in atmosphere, comfort, and convenience (pp. 25–27). 3) To retain clients and referral sources in the long run, locate in an area where you plan to be for a long time (pp. 27–28). 4) To maximize referrals, especially from indirect sources, locate within the neighborhood, city, and county areas most appealing to your desired clients (p. 28). 5) To minimize burnout, enhance future referrals, and create a stable income, before choosing your location factor in your personal and client preferences (1 and 2), rather than just the income level of residents (pp. 28–29). 6) To keep overhead low if you prefer practicing in an affluent area, choose a less expensive office that retains the features most important to you, and prioritize to reduce other practice costs (pp. 29–30).

Safety

Another important consideration in choosing an office is the general safety of the surrounding area. You may find a beautiful office that is easily affordable, but if it sits in a dangerous neighborhood, everyone could be at greater risk for crime. As always in our practices, our clients come first, especially those in psychologically vulnerable states of fear or trauma. Imagine how scary it would be for your clients to drive to an unsafe area after dark. In addition, whether working with colleagues or solo, the last thing you need is to be a sitting duck for trouble in a risky location. While you may find a great bargain in a bad area, all your rental savings (and you!) could be quickly erased in one tragic event. Even if nothing happens, you could lose considerable income if potential clients avoid your location due to safety concerns.

I will never forget how I learned about safety in one of my previous offices, in a way I hope you never do. When our building owner raised rents quite high, my colleagues, Denise, Karen, and I set out to find a new place. We were sharing expenses at the time, and wanted a space big enough so everyone could stay together. After searching around, we were pleased to find a large, reasonably priced suite in a two-story building. Driving through the area, I sensed an artistic, creative atmosphere, unique shops, and a variety of residents and visitors. The building owners weren't aware of any crime in the general area, but it was common knowledge that to the west was a less desirable part of the city.

None of us predicted what would happen later. During the next four years the unsafe area spread further east all the way to our neighborhood. Because we were all busy with our work and personal lives, we didn't really notice until it finally reached our block. A major wake-up call came from local media, who began reporting on serious crimes in the area, including rapes and assaults. At the time I had night appointments and began feeling very uneasy about seeing clients after dark. One Tuesday around 3:00 P.M. after finishing a session, I walked past the kitchen and suddenly stopped in my tracks. There on the counter was a big empty spot where the microwave had been. As my heart started racing so did I, checking each room for losses and with much relief found everything else still in its place. I quickly told Denise and Karen, and then alerted the neighbors. Everyone was stunned; no one had noticed anything suspicious on that normal business day. We also contacted the building owners and police, who responded right away.

Assessing the Safety of Potential Office Locations

I hope that in reading the lesson I learned, you will take proactive steps to avert a similar ordeal. To avoid locating in an unsafe area, first ask friends, colleagues, and other people you know for their opinions of safer versus riskier neighborhoods wherever you are looking. Then, drive around the areas you are interested in during the day and night, and on the weekend, to get your own feel for the place. Travel beyond your immediate prospective neighborhood in different directions to find out if there are any bad areas that are encroaching. Although I did drive around, it was only in the day and close to the office. If I had gone out at night and traveled further, I would have had a better sense of the place and known more accurately where unsafe areas began. With regular drives after moving in, I could have monitored these boundaries and been alerted sooner of the increasing danger.

Once you identify specific spaces you are interested in, talk with prospective office neighbors. Find out if they know of any prior safety problems in the building and your suite, and whether they feel secure working in that location. Ask whether they use their offices after usual working hours (5 or 6 P.M.) and whether the area is still safe then. When talking with our upstairs neighbors after the crime, we learned some startling information. An insurance agency had been in the building a long time, and the agency owners remembered that our very suite was burglarized more than once years ago. If we had queried them before moving in, we would have learned about this vulnerability before signing a lease.

Be sure to also ask the building owners, landlords, and/or rental agents for their knowledge of any crime history in the building and in your potential office space. Although we did ask about crime in general, we did not specifically inquire about our suite. It's certainly possible the building owners did not know or forgot about these past burglaries. But if they were aware, they would probably be more forthcoming if we explicitly asked about the space, as opposed to a general question about the area.

You can gain additional data by contacting the local police station and asking about past and current crime activity. We learned about this the hard way, too. As the police officer was completing our crime report that day, he shared his full knowledge of the same past burglaries in our suite, in addition to others that occurred recently nearby. He informed us that chronic substance abusers were most likely to blame, looking for items they could easily pawn for quick drug money. If we had contacted the local police station before committing to the office, we would have known about past crimes in advance.

In retrospect, had we taken all these steps to learn what we know now, I'm not sure whether we would have still selected the office. However, I do know I would have wanted to be more fully informed before making a decision. If we still chose to move in, we could have requested more security features, monitored the unsafe areas, and taken extra precautions on our own. Of course bad things can always happen no matter how many steps you take or how prepared you are, but the more you know and act upon that which is within your control, the better the odds of avoiding an unwanted crime.

Issue	Recommendation
Choosing a safe location for your office.	1) Ask friends, colleagues, and others you know for their opinions of the safety of areas you are considering (pp. 31–32). 2) Personally check the security of the areas you are interested in by driving around at different times; travel beyond your prospective neighborhood to discover any dangerous areas nearby (pp. 31–32). 3) After identifying specific buildings, ask your prospective office neighbors if they know of any safety problems, and whether they feel comfortable working there (pp. 31–32). 4) Ask the leasing agents for their knowledge of crime history in the building and in your specific office space (pp. 31–32). 5) For more information on crimes in the area, contact your local police station and/or research crime data from other sources (pp. 32–33).

Office Security Features

As it turned out, our trouble in that suite was not quite over. Right after the burglary, we quickly checked the office to see what additional safety features were needed. Although the front door had a deadbolt lock, the others did not. We then requested two more, one for the back door and one for the door joining the waiting room with the interior offices. Deadbolt locks are not expensive and as you can see from our experience, they are well worth the extra prevention effort. In reviewing our burglary, we further realized that even with the locks we had, we were lax during the day about locking the door separating the waiting and therapy rooms. If the door had been left unlocked that day, our burglar could have easily opened it and walked right into our private space. Always locking entryways to secure areas will go a long way to protect your space. We also ordered a low-priced, easy-to-install lock for the sliding glass window separating the waiting room from the copy and fax machines. Our burglar could have also entered this way, since the window had no lock at the time.

Unfortunately, before the deadbolt locks were installed, we were hit again, but this time apparently late at night. One morning I discovered our back door had been pried open. Almost everything of value in the office had been stolen, the copy and fax machines, and some crystal pieces from a therapy room. Luckily no one was physically victimized, our client files remained secure, and we did not have items of great value in the office to lose. However, this was our clear signal to leave the area for a safer neighborhood and office building.

After rushing to install the new locks in our current suite, we set out to find a safer office. Following the steps previously listed, we kept an eye out for an office with as much extra security as possible. As you read what we found, consider how important each safety feature is to you. Although you may not want all or even some of them, by knowing your options you can look for and choose what is most important to you.

Our first goal was to relocate away from the risky area, but within comfortable driving distance from our current office in the same city. As we had already surveyed the city in our previous office search, we quickly zeroed in on a well-known low-crime area to the east and found a building right away. The leasing agent told us the owners paid for roving security at night to periodically check the area for any suspicious activity. He did not know of any crime history in the office, building, or immediate area. He shared that there were many current tenants who saw clients at different hours, so it was unlikely that we would ever be working alone. The building was much larger than our current one, with three stories and numerous suites on each floor. We liked the idea of having many more office neighbors, further reducing our chances of being singled out for a crime. We were also pleased that the available suite was on the second floor, making it harder for a criminal to break in compared to a ground floor location. Nightlights surrounded the building outside, and there was lighted parking near the entrances and a restaurant across the street that stayed open at night.

As you consider these safety factors in your search, you may find, like we did, that choosing an office with extra security costs more. The one we were considering was fifty-five cents more per square foot than our existing office. Although we liked the added safety, we also wanted to keep overhead expenses down. Fortunately, the suite was smaller and what we gave up in space was returned in lower rent and added safety. When you are looking, remember that even if the rent is higher, you can always choose a smaller space and/or sublet to offset extra costs.

Issue	Recommendation
Ensuring the security of your building and office space.	1) To keep your clients, your office contents, and yourself safe, make sure all entryways to your office and interior rooms have locks, including deadbolts for the doors, and always use them to protect secure areas (pp. 33–34). 2) For added protection, ask the leasing agent if there is roving security or other safety measures in place for the building and your office (pp. 34–35). 3) To avoid working alone in the building, look for an arrangement where other tenants have similar hours to yours (pp. 34–35). 4) To make access more difficult for criminals, choose an office on the second floor or higher (p. 34). 5) To increase safety outside, ensure adequate night lighting around the building, entrances, and parking areas (pp. 34–35). 6) If an office with extra security costs more, keep expenses down by choosing a smaller space and/or subletting to others (p. 35). 7) For added protection, purchase a camera or other security system for your suite, or hire your own security service (pp. 35–36).

When getting to know some of our new office neighbors, Joan, a fellow therapist, confided that she was also burglarized in her previous office before moving into the same safer location and building. Her office hours extended as late as 10:00 P.M. and her suite was right down the hall. She showed us the extra security system she had purchased that visually displayed those in the waiting room. The monitor sat in the therapy room facing her and outside the client's view, so she could see anyone who came in. Depending on your needs, there are many such security measures you can take for added protection in your office. You could stick with something basic like we did and make sure deadbolt locks are on all doors, or you could buy a camera or similar video system like Joan bought. You could even hire a formal security service to install an alarm system and monitor the area.

Accessibility

Several practices will help you choose an office that is easily accessible to clients. They involve locating near freeway exits, transit stops, and selecting/arranging to provide a suitable office for clients who are disabled.

Freeways and Transit Stops

Another key feature to look for in an office is how accessible it is to clients. Buildings near freeway exits and public transportation offer easier access and, in turn, can enhance referrals and follow-throughs in ongoing treatment. Consider that saving thirty, twenty, or even ten minutes driving to a therapy appointment could really appeal to people who are already commuting a considerable distance to work or to others who are already stressed and overwhelmed by the very problems that bring them to therapy. By making their trip to see you more convenient, you take one more stressor out of their day and increase the chances they will follow through in receiving the treatment they need. Prospective clients, who search indirect referral sources such as insurance lists, yellow pages, or websites, are also more likely to select you over someone else with a less convenient office location.

My colleague, Tom, noticed this working for him firsthand when he moved his practice. His old office, although centrally located in the city, required clients to drive more surface streets for a longer time to get there. His new office was right near a freeway interchange. As soon as he moved, he began to receive remarks from continuing clients about how much easier it was to get to the new office, even though it was farther from their homes.

He also noticed an increase in new referrals, which he suspected was due in part to his new, more convenient location near the freeway exits.

Consider also that clients who do not drive may look for a therapist whose office is located near a public transportation stop. You can help these people as well as yourself by having your office close to a bus, subway, train, or other transit stop. Both of Tom's offices were near a city bus stop and some of his clients have remarked over the years that they chose to see him specifically because he was close to public transportation. Another clinician, Brian, specializes in worker's compensation evaluations and treatment. Many of his clients cannot drive and his location next to a bus stop makes it very easy for people to seek his services and follow through with ongoing care.

I have also noticed times when both new and ongoing clients were able to attend appointments because my office was near a bus stop. In one example, a new client chose me because she had lost her license for a year due to a drunk driving offense. Although she had completed an in-patient substance abuse program and was also attending AA meetings, she still had to take the bus everywhere until her license was reinstated. Other ongoing clients were able to attend appointments by taking the bus when their car broke down, when they couldn't find a ride, or after an accident when their car was being repaired. You never know what challenges clients may face in seeking help. When your office is close to public transportation, you make it easier for them to get to you no matter what happens in their lives. And you benefit as well with fewer no-shows, cancellations, and more new clients.

Handicap Access

Some of your clients may be physically challenged. By choosing a handicap accessible office, you provide a welcome option for these individuals and increase your chances that they will choose to see you. When searching, look for handicap accessibility to both the building and your office. Check your office doors to make sure someone in a wheelchair could easily pass through. See if there are clearly designated handicapped parking spots close to the building entrance. If the building is multistory, make sure it has a working elevator. Some older buildings are not handicapped accessible and have daunting steps to enter the building and to reach higher floors.

When my colleagues and I were looking for an office we were surprised how many older buildings did not have elevators or wheelchair ramps.

These options were immediately crossed off since we wanted an office accessible to clients with disabilities. The one we did choose had all the required features—handicapped parking near the entrance, a wheelchair friendly elevator, and therapy/waiting rooms large enough for a client using a wheelchair.

If you find an office that you love but it does not have disabled access, you still may be able to locate there and see handicapped clients. One possibility is to do what my colleague Sara does. She has an agreement with her therapist friend Jane, whose office is handicap accessible. If a disabled client requests Sara's services and cannot walk up the steps to her second floor office, she will sublet an hour each week from Jane in order to see her client. Although she hasn't used this option yet, she is fully prepared to do so if needed. And in the meantime, she enjoys practicing in her desired office, a beautiful older building with a unique European style.

If you don't plan to see disabled clients now, keep in mind that your practice may change over time. By having a plan to accommodate these referrals in advance, you can offer services whenever they are needed and in turn increase your clientele, a strategy that benefits everyone.

Issue	Recommendation
Choosing an office that is easily accessible to clients.	1) To provide clients easy access to your office and reduce no-shows, choose an office near freeway exits and public transportation stops (pp. 36–37). 2) To accommodate clients with handicaps and boost referrals, look for a handicap accessible building and office (pp. 37–38). 3) If you prefer an office that is not handicap accessible, sublet by the hour from a colleague who does have handicap accessibility in order to see disabled clients, or ask the building owners to add handicap accessible features (pp. 37–38).

Parking

Specific parking features are important to consider when selecting an office. They include parking availability, accessibility, and fees.

Parking Availability

An additional office feature that can be easily overlooked is parking availability. This may be especially important if you are in an urban area where many office buildings have limited spaces. Think back to a time when you couldn't find a parking space at an important event and were driving around and around in frustration, in a seemingly endless search. Now add to that the burden of, say, major depression, panic attacks, and/or agoraphobia, and this supposedly small stressor could turn into a nightmare for some of your clients. At the least this problem can increase their distress and make them late to sessions. Or instead, they could give up and drive home in even worse shape emotionally, missing important treatment.

Fortunately, you can help prevent these hardships by selecting an office with plenty of accessible parking spaces for your clients as well as for yourself. In your search, ask the building owner or leasing agent the following questions: How many parking spaces are assigned to this office? Who are the office neighbors and how many parking places are assigned to them? Are there problems at times when all spots are full? Do others inappropriately park in spaces assigned to other offices? Ask to be shown the parking lot and your designated spaces. Find out if people have experienced any safety problems when parking there, an especially important question if there is a parking garage. Later, when driving around the area in the day and night and on the weekend, check the spots to see if they are typically vacant or being used by someone else. Survey the neighborhood for high-usage buildings, such as apartment housing or popular restaurants, whose patrons might take over your parking spaces when their lots are full. Ask your prospective office neighbors for their feedback too; they may be your most accurate resources as they deal directly with parking all the time.

I learned about the importance of accessible parking firsthand in one of my previous offices. When selecting the office, my colleagues and I took what we thought was a thorough survey of available parking. The owners showed us a large parking lot in the back of the building. Four spaces were specifically assigned to our suite, and there were other guest spaces we could use as well. We figured that although four of us were sharing space, at any given time only a couple of us would be in the office at the same time, leaving two or more extra parking spaces for our clients. The office was in a mixed residential and business area, with additional street parking all around. Everything looked and sounded good, with plenty of parking options for everyone.

After moving in, all seemed fine at first. But then some clients started to mention they had a hard time finding a space, even on the street. We began to notice the area was busy most of the time, with people coming and going from the many shops and restaurants nearby. We also realized that even when just two of us were in the office, clients who arrived early for their appointments often could not find any open spaces. Between our current clients and us, our designated spots were taken and often the guest spaces were, too. Perhaps if we had checked to see whether parking spaces were available when driving around the area, we would have seen this problem earlier.

On top of that, our residential neighbors would often park their cars in our spaces overnight, leaving them there during daytime business hours. Sometimes we got so frustrated that we had these vehicles towed, but this took a lot of time and effort, and was not a productive use of our limited resources. If we had kept an eye open for high-usage buildings in our earlier drives, we might have noticed the lack of designated parking spaces for the renters in the multiunit apartment buildings right behind our parking lot.

In addition, at certain times during the week every possible parking space was taken. When we asked our office neighbors why, we learned that the insurance company upstairs had regular meetings with all their agents, including those who normally worked in the field. If we had talked with our neighbors about parking before moving in, we would have learned about these gatherings, the lack of spaces, and the renters who left their cars at all hours.

Parking Accessibility and Fees

Find out if there are any parking fees and/or gates to navigate. You can ask the leasing agent, your office neighbors, and look around for parking meters, payment kiosks, or automatic gates. Free, open parking may be important to stressed-out clients who do not want to pay another fee or cross a barrier in order to see you. If there is an expensive parking garage, you could negotiate with the owner or manager for reduced fee parking for your clients. Although you may be told no, the potential savings to your clients are well worth the effort in asking. When prospective clients call to learn about my services, I always mention the free parking at my office and they almost always react very positively to this news. Although this may not solely determine whether someone picks you over another therapist, it can definitely be a perk for those clients who do see you.

Issue	Recommendation
Considering specific parking features, such as, availability, accessibility, and fees.	1) To assess parking at prospective offices, ask the leasing agent and your office neighbors about parking availability and over usage problems (pp. 39–40). 2) To discover potential parking problems, check whether your prospective parking spaces are usually full during your drives around the area (pp. 39–40). 3) To compare parking challenges and costs, check for automated parking barriers and fees (p. 40).

Specific Office Features: Utilities

Specific features of utilities and cleaning services are also importat to compare before selecting your office. They include additional fees, utility hours, temperature controls, and restrooms.

Utility and Cleaning Service Fees

In addition to rental expense, any office you choose could have separate monthly utility or cleaning fees. These potential costs could really add up, so it's in your best interest to learn about extra fees before you commit to a space. To find out, ask your leasing agent the following questions: Is there a separate utility fee? How much is it? Is there a cleaning service? Do they clean individual offices? What specifically do they clean? Does this service require an extra fee? Add any fees to your monthly budget planning, so you can accurately compare total expenses for each office you are considering.

For many therapists I know, utilities and cleaning services are included in their rent. This is true for me, but this wasn't always the case. In a previous office, each therapist paid fifty dollars each month for cleaning services alone. We were also assessed an additional utility fee each month. In choosing the new office, although the rent per square foot was higher, the savings from no extra cleaning or utility fees completely offset this cost.

Utility Hours

If your practice hours extend beyond normal business hours, it will be important to make sure all utilities operate whenever you are in the office. Some office buildings turn these off at a set time, and if you don't know this, you could find yourself in a freezing or sweltering office after hours.

To prevent this hardship, before committing to a lease agreement, specifically ask if the utilities shut off at certain hours. If you find an office you
love with this problem, ask the leasing agent for adjustments to keep utilities on in your space. Be sure to negotiate utility hours before signing a
lease so you can factor this information into your decision about whether
or not to sign a lease.

Temperature Controls

When discussing utilities, also find out where the temperature controls are
for your space. Ideally you want them to be in your office, so you can
adjust the air whenever needed to fit your preference. However, sometimes
suites are heated and cooled in groups, and the thermostat may not be in
your office. This can create quite a problem if your neighbors like it cool
and you like it warmer, or if the air is distributed unevenly among the
rooms. To identify any potential problems before you commit to a space,
ask the leasing agent, your immediate office neighbors, and, when possible, the past tenants if they know of any such temperature troubles. If so,
and you like everything else about that office, you may be able to work
something out before committing to the space in order to prevent similar
temperature problems.

My office neighbor, Melanie, learned about this after moving in down
the hall. She hadn't asked these questions beforehand, but quickly noticed
how cold it was in her suite. She tried to adjust the thermostat on her wall
but it didn't seem to help. In talking with the building manager, she
learned that the air in her office was actually controlled through the thermostat in the office next door. He suggested she talk with these neighbors—an attorney and his staff—which she did. She learned that much of
the time no one was there because the attorney was often in a trial. Additionally, any adjustments didn't seem to affect his office temperature much
either way. He suggested that she could come into his suite anytime to
adjust the thermostat, and even gave her a set of keys to use when they
were not there. What could have been a very stressful issue for Melanie
turned out to be workable, since her office neighbors were so helpful. If
something like this happens to you, your neighbors may not be so accommodating. By asking questions ahead of time, you can identify and hopefully remedy problems before moving in, saving you and your clients
discomfort and stress.

Restrooms

Another important office feature to check on is where the restrooms are and how convenient they will be without interfering with your work. This may be especially important if you and your clients use the facilities often. Some offices have a restroom in the suite, which could be either very convenient or disruptive to a therapy session. To find out ahead of time, test to see if noise from the restroom would carry over to the therapy room(s). Other offices may have restrooms that are hard to access, taking longer to find and cutting into scheduled time. Be sure to discuss this issue with the leasing agent to come up with solutions to possible problems before these issues surface.

In my practice, the facilities are used a lot. Having a restroom conveniently located down the hall, outside the suite itself, has been a great plus for everyone. For easy access, clients use a key that is placed in the waiting room, returning it when they are done. For extra protection, the key has a large wooden attachment to prevent clients from accidentally putting it in their purse or pocket. To avoid any awkward moments of bumping into a client in the restroom, I also use this "client" key instead of my own.

Issue	Recommendation
Comparing utilities and cleaning services when selecting your office.	1) To survey each prospective office, ask your leasing agent about utilities and cleaning fees and services; to accurately compare office expenses, add extra fees to your monthly rent estimates (p. 41). 2) To assess whether utilities will stay on if you plan to work beyond business hours, discuss and confirm solutions in advance with the leasing agent (p. 41–42). 3) To compare heating/cooling systems, ask prospective neighbors and past tenants if they know of any problems; find out also where the temperature controls are located (p. 42). 4) If you learn of any utility system problems, negotiate solutions with the leasing agent before committing to the space (pp. 41–42). 5) Check the restroom locations, looking for accessibility, convenience, and minimal disruption to therapy sessions (p. 43).

Lease, Size, and Preferences

Several additional features are important to consider before selecting your office. They include lease length, a sublease option, office size and preferences, and desired changes.

Lease Length

Another important factor in selecting your office is the length of your lease. Ideally the shortest commitment will give you the most flexibility to move your office quickly, if necessary, without financial consequences. However, this benefit may be offset by a greater possibly of rent increases each time your lease is renewed. To help in deciding what's best for you, after finding out the lease length, ask the agent and your prospective office neighbors how often rents have been raised in the past few years, and what kinds of increases are expected in future years. If the rent is not likely to be raised very often, a shorter lease may be more appealing. Estimate how long you are likely to practice in the office, and if you share space with others, ask them how long they plan to stay. If everyone expects to remain a long time, a longer lease may work well.

If you are just getting started, favor a shorter lease at first to protect yourself financially. If your practice does not build quickly enough to cover expenses when the lease expires, you will then be able to choose a different arrangement without being stuck in a long, financially draining contract. As detailed in Chapter 1, you could then consider less costly practice options such as subletting, expense sharing, or joining a group.

My current office lease is month-to-month, and so far the rent has increased once in four years. The short lease length was very appealing after committing to a four-year contract in a previous location. In that office, three of us shared rent and about the time one therapist left, a new one moved in, keeping the rent payments covered the entire time. We were very lucky that we lasted the whole length of the lease without having to pay extra rent for someone who left without a replacement.

Sublease Option

Another important feature to look for in a lease is the option to sublease the office to someone else. This will give you the most flexibility in your office arrangement, allowing you to work solo or with others whenever you desire. For example, if you start out solo but discover that your income does not cover overhead costs as much as you'd like, you could sublet space to lower your rent payment and automatically boost your return. Or, if you are in full-time practice and decide to reduce to part-time, you could rent the office during the time you'll be away and keep overhead low as you lighten your client load. Whatever your practice needs, the subleasing option will allow you to accommodate your changing preferences.

Office Size

When choosing your office, you can keep expenses down by only paying for the space you need. Rents tend to go up and not down over the years; you can minimize this added outlay by keeping your office size to only what you will use. Review your practice needs ahead of time. If you see groups, families, or couples you may need a larger therapy room than if you were working exclusively with individuals. If you see children, you may need extra space for play therapy. If you do not currently work with these populations but would like to in the future, it can help to estimate your practice needs in the next few years to choose the best space for now and also plan for later.

If you are concerned with clients' reactions to a small space, remember that they are motivated to see you primarily for your services. Although of course you want a clean, professional looking office, you may be surprised to find that clients care a lot less than you do about specific features such as size. When moving to my current office, I was also concerned that clients might react negatively to the new, smaller therapy room. Their reaction was just the opposite of what I feared; clients commented positively on the change and no one expressed discontent with the smaller space. Since I currently see individuals only and do not anticipate seeing families or larger groups, this space works well for my practice and is very cost-effective. By renting only what you need, you can enjoy savings without compromising client appeal.

Office Preferences

You may also have special preferences when considering prospective offices. Certain features may be very important (e.g., a window with a pleasant view); others may be deal breakers, such as outside traffic noise or disruptive office neighbors. When deciding what you do and do not want, ask yourself the following sample questions which you can modify to fit your individual preferences. Is there a window in the therapy room? If so, what is the view? Are there any people or activities nearby that could disrupt therapy sessions? Who are the immediate office neighbors next door, and above or below? Does their work involve activities, noises, or smells that could disrupt therapy? Where is the office located in the building? Is there a nearby elevator, restroom, or frequently used stairwell that could be disruptive? Does noise from outside traffic pose a problem? These things may not be immediately apparent when you are looking, but some could turn into significant office stressors. By asking the leasing agent, your prospective office neighbors, and, if possible, past tenants these questions ahead of time, you will have a good idea what to expect if you decide on the space.

After moving to a new office, my colleague, Jennifer, discovered many of these issues quite by surprise. Although she made sure the office had a window with a pretty view of trees, other unexpected issues became obvious over time. The office was located in the back of the building on the second floor and she soon discovered that you could hear people walking up and down the stairs nearby. Her immediate neighbor to the right had a booming voice and when he met with clients, sometimes his discussions carried into the therapy room. The upstairs neighbor was a fellow therapist and at times, usually late in the evening, she could hear footsteps above. The trash bin was below the office on the ground floor and every Tuesday was collected, sometimes disturbing her in the middle of relaxation exercises with clients.

While none of these issues alone was enough for Jennifer to consider leaving, in combination they did make doing therapy more stressful. Finding out about these components of office selection ahead of time can help you know what's in store, so you can address any major problems in advance, or move on to another office if there are too many negative features.

When Denise, Karen, and I were looking for an office, the leasing agent of a building we were considering told us about the neighboring hair and nail salon on the ground floor. He disclosed that the past tenants in the upstairs suite we were looking at had left in part because of the strong, unpleasant smells drifting up from below. He also pointed out the location of a dentist's office right next door, sharing that through one adjoining wall you could hear the whirring noise of a drill whenever it was turned on. Based on these features alone, we decided to move on in our search. When you are looking, your leasing agent may not be so forthcoming. By also querying office neighbors and past tenants, and checking these issues out in person, you can make sure you are fully informed when choosing your own office.

Office Changes

You may also prefer to make changes to an office you are considering. For example, you might want new carpet, blinds, paint, extra locks, a wall moved, an extra door, or other changes to fit your practice. To ensure this happens before moving in, first survey the space to decide what changes you want. Then, ask the leasing agent for these accommodations before signing a lease. If your requests are granted, put them in writing and have them signed along with projected dates of completion for extra assurance. If you do not get what you want, you still have time to decide whether to accept the office as is, or move on to another one that is more accommodating to your preferences.

Before committing to a previous office, my colleagues and I requested that the suite be configured completely differently. We wanted three large therapy rooms, a kitchen/conference room, a business office area, and a smaller waiting room. To our surprise, we learned that the building owners did their own carpentry work. They agreed to rebuild the office suite to our specifications, and also installed new carpet and flooring that we had selected. In addition, we were able to wallpaper our therapy rooms however we wanted. Our only extra fees were for an extra door we requested, leading from the kitchen to the outside parking lot, and for extra soundproofing in the walls.

We chose this office in large part because the owners agreed in writing to fulfill our multiple requests before moving in. When you are considering what you would like in your prospective offices, be sure to ask for *all* the changes you want first, before committing to a lease. As we were surprised to find out, you may just get everything you request; or, you could receive a majority of things you want. However, if you don't ask you will never know, and you will be forgoing an opportune time to negotiate preferred changes.

As you decide on an office, researching and comparing the important features of location, safety, accessibility, expenses, and specific features, can help you to quickly size up the situation in each prospective office. By attending to these issues as you choose, you can increase your happiness at work, deliver better services, bring in more clients, reduce overhead, and increase income all at the same time. Certain factors may be more or less important to you depending on your specific practice needs, and may not by themselves determine your office preference. However, knowing this information ahead of time will help you weigh the pros and cons and avoid any unforeseen surprises once you choose an office and begin practicing. If you find any problems, you will be able to proactively address them before committing to a lease or move on to another office with the features you want.

Issue	Recommendation
Comparing lease features, office size, and preferences when selecting your office.	1) To choose the best lease length, consider how often rents are raised, and how long you (and your colleagues) plan to stay in the office (pp. 44–45). 2) To protect yourself financially when getting started in practice, choose a short lease (pp. 44–45). 3) To provide the most flexibility in arranging your office, make sure your lease contract includes the option to sublease (pp. 44–45). 4) To keep overhead expense low, review your practice needs in advance and rent only the space you will use (p. 45). 5) To compare office features and potential stressors, ask the leasing agent, office neighbors, and past tenants questions modified to fit your preferences (pp. 45–46). 6) To ensure desired office changes, identify and confirm everything you want done in writing before signing a lease (pp. 47–48).

CHAPTER THREE

Selecting a Cost-Effective Communication System

A good communications system is an essential element of every private practice. It can also be a considerable expense. By carefully assessing your needs, comparing features, and paying for only what is necessary, you can greatly reduce this monthly expense by setting up and maintaining your own system. With lower costs, your net earnings (income minus expenses) will automatically increase. Regardless of the number of clients you see, this extra return will help stabilize and preserve your income, especially during slow times. Your clients will benefit too, as you become less worried about your bottom line and more able to focus on providing quality care. They will also appreciate immediate, direct contact, especially during critical times.

Large Group Practices

Practice groups employing full-time secretaries were fairly common before the 1990s, when managed care insurance began to reduce fees and limit networks. Back then, when reimbursements were much higher, groups could more easily pay employee salaries and still net a strong profit. However, according to the October, 2000, *Psychotherapy Finances* Fee, Practice, and Managed Care Survey, group practices spent 34.7 percent of their gross revenue on expenses, a 3 percent increase compared to three years earlier. Combine these added costs with the 15 percent fee reductions from managed care reimbursement detailed by the same survey, and a full-time secretary's salary could eat up a much larger portion of net income than ever before.

If you are in a group practice experiencing such a financial struggle, your group could reduce costs significantly by replacing secretarial and/or contracted answering services with individual phone lines and voicemail messaging. Voicemail can be set up through the phone lines, cellular phones, or pagers. Therapists can make calls at work from their individual phone lines, and calls away from the office using, home, other land line, and/or cellular phones. If a central number is preferred to advertise to clients, one phone line can use voicemail or an answering machine, playing a greeting message stating every member's name, specialties, and separate contact number.

These systems offer streamlined communication while saving you hundreds (compared to an answering service) or even thousands (compared to a secretary) of dollars per month. Our unique field of mental health is also replete with privacy concerns and delicate, complicated therapeutic issues. When clients call, therapists frequently need to directly respond to them anyway, often making an office staff unnecessary. By eliminating this intermediary, clients gain faster, more efficient communication, and you save the cost of extraneous services.

Changes to office staff may be easier to incorporate if group members are already responsible for other practice tasks, such as scheduling and record keeping. Some group members may be ambivalent about becoming their own secretary. However, once procedures and policies are in place, they will find it surprisingly easy to handle their own calls, schedule appointments, and even take care of other office management tasks, such as verifying insurance and billing.

The practice where I started was a typical example of a group with a high communications expense. It was a large, multi-specialty group with two full-time secretaries and an answering system for after-hour calls. Everyone in the practice listed one central office phone number as their contact number. When clients called, they talked with a secretary who screened calls, routed messages to therapists, and performed other tasks during business hours. Each clinician also had an individual emergency pager, allowing clients to call and leave a message 24 hours-a-day. Although these services worked fine, they also added to overhead expenses. Whatever the level of gross earnings, these costs predictably reduced net profit every month. I remember working in this group and receiving messages that were simply passed on from clients to the secretary to me. It seemed a waste of resources and time to pay someone to do this when people could directly leave a message at my individual contact number.

In this group and others like it, expenses could be greatly reduced by eliminating the secretaries and answering system and instead using individual phone lines and messaging systems to make and receive calls. If a group prefers to have an office manager, a direct communication system would reduce the secretary's workload, as therapists respond to their own phone calls. With a smaller workload, the office manager could complete remaining office tasks more quickly, and secretarial hours could be reduced, lowering the expense for this outside service.

Small Expense-Sharing Groups

Small expense-sharing group arrangements are common these days, where a few full- or part-time therapists share office space. In these groups, in which individuals often take care of their own practices, these suggested communication methods may be easy to implement. Individual systems also provide easier expense tracking and payment, as each person can receive and pay bills independently.

My friend, Laura, discovered the value of streamlining communications systems when sharing an office suite with two other therapists. She joined this small group after they had already been in practice for a few years. Although there was no secretary in the suite, there was a multiline phone system that had been used for years. Four total phone lines were connected, one for each therapist and the fourth dedicated to the fax machine. One phone number was advertised to the public and when prospective clients called, this phone line was connected to an answering machine whose message directed the caller to each therapist's individual pager number.

This arrangement worked fine until the multiline phone system broke, and the phone specialist informed them of the high cost to repair or replace this expensive, complicated system. He suggested an alternative of using individual phone lines, which would eliminate extra fees for new equipment or custom installation. The group quickly decided on these less

expensive phone lines, which also simplified client access to each therapist. They eliminated the central phone number, answering machine, and
cumbersome message referring callers to separate numbers. Instead, each
therapist offered her individual pager number as the contact for clients,
allowing them to directly leave a voice message at the first number they
call. As Laura found out, by evaluating your group situation and looking
for ways to simplify and reduce communication costs, you can provide
easier access for clients and lower overhead at the same time.

Issue	Recommendation
Reducing communications expenses in group arrangements.	1) To keep costs low and streamline communications, choose individual phone lines and voicemail messaging over expensive secretarial and/or outside answering services (pp. 49–51). 2) If your group prefers an office manager, to reduce his/her workload, have therapists handle their own calls; as remaining office tasks are finished sooner, expensive secretarial hours can be reduced (pp. 50–51). 3) To provide efficient, direct access for clients, eliminate multiline phone systems, central phone numbers, and messages referring callers to separate numbers (pp. 51–52).

Expense-Sharing with One Colleague

Another way to cut communication expenses is to share the same office
space with someone. This can work well if you each work part-time and
can alternate use of the same space. In addition to splitting rent, you can
cut phone bills in half by sharing the same service. If you each work at different times, you can use just one phone line, saving the cost of installation and monthly service for additional lines. A phone can be placed in
the therapy room for outgoing calls, with the ringer turned off during sessions to prevent interruptions. Individual messaging systems set up
through a pager or cellular phone can provide direct access for clients, pre-
cluding the need for a separate answering machine or incoming voice messages on the telephone line. The fax machine can be hooked up to the

same telephone line, listed publicly as the fax number. If you have a supply room, business machine area, or other private, secure space outside the therapy room, you can place it there to avoid disturbances from incoming faxes. In this way, if your office mate ever comes to the office needing to make a call while you are in session, he/she could use the readily available fax phone.

I can attest to this working well from my own shared office experience. My colleague Denise and I rented a suite that included a waiting room, a supply room, and a therapy room. We agreed upon an alternating schedule, each working in the office two days weekly. Since only one of us was there at a time, we split the cost of one phone line, placing a phone in the therapy room and the fax machine in the supply room, each connected to separate phone jacks. Clients directly called our pager numbers to leave messages, and we returned calls at work using the fax/phone line. I remember many times when one of us would stop by the office when the other was in session. Having the fax machine in the supply room was very convenient; we could check faxes and make calls using the fax phone without disturbing ongoing therapy in the other room. On rare occasions, if one of us came in when the other was on the phone, we could make calls with our cellular phones, which we carried at all times.

In addition to serving as a possible messaging system, cell phones provide a convenient, portable method by which to call clients whenever you are away from a land line. Although most people already have a cellular phone, if you do not, it is recommended as a good supplemental communications system for your practice. However, for reasons detailed later, cellular service is not recommended as a primary communications system.

Eliminating Office Telephone Service

If the volume of calls is small at your practice site, you could consider downsizing even more by completely eliminating telephone service at work. Instead you could use a cellular phone at work plus your home or other telephone when away from the office, increasing your monthly savings. A paging or cellular service could comprise your public contact number, answering system, and paging all in one for a very reasonable fee. If you frequently change practice locations or affiliations, you also save the cost of installation fees by forgoing phone service.

This option is more feasible if you practice part-time, do not need a phone line for other activities, and/or are away from your office regularly. One way to determine low call volume is if all your calls at the office could be handled through your cellular phone alone. To check, average monthly minutes used from two or more recent office telephone bills, add this to your typical cellular minutes used, and see if the total fits within a reasonably priced monthly cellular service plan.

If you need a publishable number at which to receive faxes, you will need to keep a regular telephone line. However, if your volume of faxes is low and you could eliminate a public fax number, you could send faxes from a home or other secure machine and arrange on a case-by-case basis to receive them the same way. You would just need to inform senders that the fax transmission is for one time only and it is not a regular fax line, if that is the case.

If you use your home line for faxes, do not use it with clients, even if you present it as a fax line only. This preserves your privacy and an important boundary, ensuring clients will not have your number or give it to anyone else. Clients in distress who have your number could easily forget it is a fax line and call at any time, destroying your privacy and creating much stress for you. If you don't have another secure fax line to use, you could exchange information with clients through the mail or in person at your office.

Another issue to consider before canceling office telephone service is that you will not be able to continue complimentary yellow and white pages as well as 411 listings. See page 61 for a detailed discussion of this issue to help in your decision.

Issue	Recommendation
Reducing communications expenses by sharing or removing telephone service.	1) To cut phone bills in half, alternate usage of the same space and phone line with a colleague (pp. 52–53). 2) For greater savings, if compatible with your practice needs, eliminate a telephone line at work and instead use a cellular phone for calls; arrange for secure faxes on a case-by-case basis (pp. 52–53). 3) To preserve the privacy of your home phone number, do not use your home line for client faxes; instead use another secure fax line, mail, or in-person options to exchange information (p. 54).

Cellular Phone Service

After reading the previous suggestions, you might be thinking, why not just use a cellular phone as my contact number for voicemail, paging, and for all my calls? No need for any phone lines, pager fees, or extra equipment purchases. At first this sounds very efficient and cost effective—one full-service system in a small phone you can carry all the time. Although you may choose it for your messaging system and some professional calls, before opting exclusively for a cell phone in your practice, first consider the following questions and issues.

Are you concerned about the increased risk of poor reception and dropped calls? Cellular connections are much more likely to experience these problems than land connections. Factor in the fragile emotional status of many clients seeking help, and a dropped call, frustrating echo, or static on the line could quickly trigger significant distress. At the least, these annoyances convey a less-than-professional image, something to avoid whenever possible.

Is reduced privacy during calls a concern? Many extremely sensitive and serious issues are a normal part of everyday therapy practice. Clients often share with us issues, such as affairs, addictions, unwanted pregnancies, plans to leave an abusive marriage, etc. they would be horrified if anyone else knew. In wireless communication, as opposed to land phone lines, there is less certainty of being able to honor client confidentiality during such critical and revealing calls.

Are you concerned about receiving calls at inappropriate times, such as when you are having lunch with a friend or sitting on a bus? Unless you rigorously remember to turn your cellular phone off when you are not prepared to take calls, you run the risk of receiving calls at improper times.

Do you need a publishable number to receive faxes and/or do you want dial up Internet access at work? If so, you will need a telephone line for these activities.

Do you want a courtesy yellow/white pages listing to advertise your services? When paying for a phone line you automatically get free listings in these directories. You also have the option of upgrading to larger yellow page ads at a discount. If you do not have a phone line, you will need to pay to be included in these directories (see p. 61).

Will your call volume be high? All cellular calls are charged whether you make or receive them and the fees can quickly add up this way. For example, if you average ten professional calls daily at just two minutes per call, working five days a week, you are using 100 minutes a week and 450 minutes a month. Double your daily calls to twenty or call length to four minutes and monthly usage jumps to 900 minutes. And these totals do not include additional personal calls. Although cellular calling plans may advertise thousands of minutes for a reasonable price, the majority of included time is often during night and weekend hours. Calls made outside the allowed timeframe, typically during business hours when you would use the most minutes, are charged a separate and much higher fee. These charges can quickly add up if your only communications system is a cellular phone.

Will you be calling many toll-free and local numbers? These calls are either free or minimally charged by telephone companies. In contrast, every cell phone call is charged, no matter whom you call. Many insurance companies have toll-free numbers and when calling them, you will more than likely be placed on hold. When using a phone line, you will save on these calls, no matter how long you must wait to get through.

Will you be using a toll-free contact number? If so, you can only get these through regular telephone or pager services, as cellular phones do not support 800 numbers.

If you answer yes to one or more of these questions, you should use a land line telephone in addition to cellular service. A phone line can circumvent these cellular phone problems and be cost effective too.

Issue	Recommendation
Having cellular service as your only communication system can be problematic.	1) For the best transmission quality and most privacy, use a telephone line whenever possible to call clients (p. 55). 2) If you need any of the following—a public fax number, dial-up Internet access at work, courtesy yellow/white pages listings, and/or a toll-free contact number—consider a telephone line for your office, which will allow for these activities (pp. 55–56). 3) To keep cellular costs down, use a telephone line when possible for high volume, toll-free, and local calls (pp. 55–56).

Messaging System Options

Depending on your practice needs and preferences, you can set up a messaging system through a telephone line, cellular phone, or pager. Each method has benefits and drawbacks, so carefully consider these factors before choosing your system. Your decision will also determine where your public work number originates, so it's in your best interest to use the same method as long as possible. Although you could change to a different system later on, this may require changing public contact numbers, creating more expense and work for you in notifying everyone of the new number. For example, you could access your voice mail through an answering service, but as the three methods mentioned above are the top choices offering streamlined communication at a low cost, we will focus on these.

Telephone Line

Your first messaging option is through a telephone line. You could use a voicemail system, which most phone companies include in monthly service plans at no extra cost, or you could purchase a separate answering machine and hook it up yourself. If you plan to have a phone line at work, either of these two options could be cost effective and efficient. However, your better choice is usually telephone voicemail, which generally offers more calling features and convenience. Whatever message system you select will automatically record incoming messages and give you the option to answer calls directly whenever you are free. All you need to do is record a greeting and set the number of rings before the system automatically answers.

Call Forwarding

If you choose one of these two phone message systems, in order to receive calls immediately when you are away from the office, forward calls to another phone line, a cellular phone, pager, or periodically call in for messages. Your phone company may even offer a pager and paging service you can add to your phone line for an additional monthly cost. If you work with clients at high risk for crises, your response time to calls could be critical in preventing harm. If you are not alerted of your messages right away, you could miss the chance to intervene and be faced with a tragic result later. You could also lose new client referrals to other clinicians who answer their calls right away.

Most telephone service plans include this call-forwarding feature at no extra cost. Some answering machines also have this call-forwarding capability. When forwarding calls to another phone messaging system, be sure to record another professional greeting on that phone for callers to hear. In contrast, with pager or cellular phone messaging systems, you don't have to forward messages from a phone line or record additional greetings on different phones. Instead, all calls are streamlined to one place.

Other Factors to Consider

If you are considering a phone line messaging option, find out whether voicemail, call forwarding, and/or paging are included with your telephone service. If not, ask how expensive they are to add, so you can compare costs with other messaging options. Find out if incoming calls are automatically forwarded to your voicemail if the line is being used. Then, if you are using the line, incoming callers will still be able to leave messages and no calls will be lost. If you prefer an answering machine, look for one that includes a call-forwarding feature. With answering machines, as opposed to telephone voicemail, automatic recording of messages may not be possible if you are using the line.

If your service includes a call-waiting feature, consider forgoing this option altogether or deactivating it before every call to a client. Do this also with any other phone you use to call clients. Interruptions during phone calls can be very irritating and distracting to your clients as well as yourself, especially during intense, emotionally-charged crisis calls.

If you plan on heavy fax or Internet usage, you may need a separate line for these activities. Otherwise, a busy line could block incoming faxes and you may not receive immediate alerts of important calls while you are using the line. One way to avoid paying for another line is to use alternative cellular or paging messaging options for incoming calls.

Next, ask yourself if you plan to share telephone service with one or more colleagues. If so, and you are individual practitioners sharing the same messaging system, privacy violations are likely when clients leave messages. In addition, if a member of the group changes affiliations in the future, you will have to decide who keeps the contact number and who must go to the trouble of changing to a new one. To prevent these problems, you would each need to pay for separate telephone lines, adding an expense for service you will not fully use. A better choice in this case is an individual paging or cellular service messaging option, preserving privacy, contact numbers, and savings.

Another point to consider is whether your practice hours will be full-time, part-time, or variable. You may want to stop or start telephone service depending on your current situation, to avoid paying for service you don't use or resume service you need. If you set up a contact number through your phone line, it will be a lot of work to switch your number and messaging system if you stop service in the future. If your number is through paging or cellular service, you can keep the same contact number whether you have telephone service or not.

If you plan to work part-time in different locations, you may also want different contact numbers for each area. However, multiple telephone lines quickly become expensive, and you end up paying for much more service than you will use. With a paging service, you can get more than one contact number linked to your pager for a small, additional monthly fee.

One fellow practitioner who chose a telephone messaging system is Paula, whose story you already know. To streamline her practice, she switched to this system from an expensive outside answering service and it works well for her. She is in full-time solo practice in one office, has one telephone line, and uses the voicemail included in her monthly service. Although her phone company offers paging service for an extra fee, instead she uses her free voicemail call-forwarding feature. When away from the office she forwards calls to the telephone line where she'll be, usually at home. She recorded the same voicemail greeting on her office, home, and other lines, so when office messages are forwarded callers always hear her professional greeting.

If Paula is away from a land line, she calls her office voicemail for messages frequently, ensuring a quick response to calls. She also uses the office line for occasional faxes, directing people to call first before sending them, allowing her to connect the fax machine for transmission. This strategy saves her the cost of another fax line. She has saved hundreds each month compared to what an answering service would cost, and her clients enjoy much better communication with her now. She no longer has to worry about answering service employees making mistakes or dropping calls, something she says happened much too often with the old service.

Paging Service or Cellular Phone

Two other options to consider for your messaging system are a paging service or cellular phone. These are inexpensive, efficient, portable, and solve many potential problems in using telephone service for incoming calls. For a rea-

Issue	Recommendation
Considering a telephone line with voicemail as your messaging system.	1) For cost-effective telephone messaging, use the voicemail included with the service or an external answering machine; to immediately receive calls, use call forwarding when away from the office (pp. 57–58). 2) To compare telephone costs with other messaging options, price fees for calling features; to prevent dropped messages, verify that incoming calls are forwarded to voicemail if your line is being used (p. 58). 3) To prevent incoming fax/message delays, use a separate line for heavy fax or Internet usage; for the most savings, choose a paging or cellular option instead of an additional telephone line as your messaging system (p. 58.) 4) Other reasons to consider paging or cellular messaging: • If you plan to share telephone service with a colleague. • If your practice hours may change in the future. • If you work part-time in different locations (pp. 58–59).

sonable monthly fee you get voicemail, message alerts, and a phone number to advertise as your work number. By carrying the pager or phone at all times, you can receive direct, immediate alerts whenever calls are received. You can then return calls from any phone you choose. If you use a telephone line for faxes, Internet, and/or return calls, there will be no interference problems with incoming calls because they will come in on a completely different system. If you change your practice hours or work affiliations, you can keep the same low-cost pager or cell service and contact number. And now, if you change service companies, you can keep your same number.

Issues to Consider Before Choosing

There are disadvantages to consider with these choices as well, however. As mentioned, with wireless service, you may experience more transmission and privacy problems than with land line calls. One way to reduce this problem is to return client calls from telephone lines whenever possible.

You can increase privacy even more during land line calls by using corded phones instead of cordless ones.

Another potential problem arises if you want to list your pager or cellular number in the phone directories and with 411; as I stated earlier, you may have to pay a monthly charge for this service. When using local land line phone service you typically get complimentary listings in these directories. If you plan to have a telephone line for other activities outside of a messaging system (e.g., for faxes, Internet, return calls), you may be able to avoid a charge by substituting your wireless number in these free listings. If you don't have a telephone line, you will be charged to place pager or cellular numbers in directory listings. To find out for sure, call your phone company ahead of time before choosing your messaging system. Start by calling the number for business service and discuss these scenarios and potential fees with someone in the directories department.

If the fees are large and directory listings are important to you, you may want to stick with a telephone line messaging system and avoid this extra expense. If you plan to rely on the yellow pages for a majority of referrals, this issue will be crucial. Directory listings provide a professional image and immediate access to anyone, including new and returning clients as well as referring colleagues. In my practice, a small but significant number of new clients find me in the yellow pages. Other returning clients have told me they checked the phone book to make sure I was still in practice. And some have found me in the directory after losing my number or address.

However, if listing fees are high and you don't plan to rely on phone directories for referrals, you could opt out of these listings and still pursue a paging or cellular messaging option. With the increase in Internet usage, there are now many ways to list your services in addition to phone books. If you contract with insurance companies or become a member of any professional organizations, your practice will probably be listed for free on their Internet websites. If they print directories for members, you will be listed in those as well. Clients may also find you through toll-free referral lines offered through their insurance carriers. You could even set up your own Internet website and/or list your services with various Internet therapy directories. With the increase in such alternative advertising, you may find yourself less in need of a phone listing.

Another problem with cellular messaging occurs if you use it for both business and personal calls and always answer immediately. In doing this you are more likely to blur personal and professional boundaries because you lose a layer of privacy and screening of calls that you would have with a separate system for business messages only. One way to reduce this problem is to use your cell phone like a pager; record a professional greeting, never answer calls directly, and instead listen to voicemail messages as soon as they are received. Screening your calls allows you to decide when and where to return them, rather than remain immediately available anytime someone wants to talk. You could tell family and friends of this change, assuring them that you will return their calls after they leave voice messages. If your service includes caller ID, you could also screen calls visually, answering personal calls after recognizing phone numbers of family and friends.

As you consider this option, remember that cellular calls during business hours can get expensive, especially if you exceed calling plan limits. If you expect to have high call volume, this choice may turn out to be more costly than paging messaging. Other disadvantages are that you are only allowed one number per cellular phone, and if you change to a new number you cannot have a forwarding message directing callers to the new number.

Another therapist I know, Judy, uses her cellular phone as a messaging system and it works well for her. She works part-time in more than one office and is not sure how long she will stay in these arrangements working with her current associates. Her goal is to increase her clientele and eventually transition to full-time solo practice in her own office in the same general area. She uses her cellular voicemail to receive messages and has recorded a professional greeting for all callers to hear. She normally uses the phone as a pager, to automatically record new messages and alert her after they arrive. If she answers the phone directly, she assumes it is a professional call and greets callers accordingly. She tries to return most of her calls through land line phones to avoid privacy and transmission problems, and to keep cell costs low. When working at her part-time offices, she pays a small monthly fee to use phone lines there. When at home she uses the phone line there. When away from a land line, she returns calls on her cellular phone.

Benefits of Paging Service

The paging system option—my personal preference—offers solutions to many cellular messaging problems. Since you won't be directly answering calls, you have a built-in layer of privacy and screening. By designating your pager exclusively for incoming business calls, you can still use your cellular phone for personal calls and eliminate any blurring of personal and professional boundaries. You also pay one low fee monthly, typically much cheaper than cellular rates. And you have the option of adding more than one number to your paging service for a small additional monthly charge. For example, my company charges just two dollars more per month for an additional number. In contrast, you are only allowed one number per cellular phone and telephone line; if you want more you will need to pay for separate service at a substantial fee for each additional number.

One situation where you may want extra contact numbers is if you practice in two or more places and want to add a number for each separate location. Companies will typically allow up to five numbers at the same additional low fee for each one, receiving all calls through the same paging system. You could also use a separate number for emergencies like my colleague Bill does. He has two numbers, the first for a general greeting that includes a directive to call the second number in the event of an emergency. That way, when he is paged he will know if the call is an emergency by the number flashing on his pager screen. If it is his first number, he knows it is a routine call; if the second shows up, he knows it is an emergency that he must respond to immediately.

Issue	Recommendation
Considering a paging service or cellular phone for your messaging system.	1) To reduce transmission and privacy problems with wireless systems, return client calls from telephone lines using corded phones whenever possible (pp. 59–60). 2) Before choosing a system, ask the phone company about fees to list non-phone numbers; if you plan a phone line for other uses (e.g., fax, Internet) ask to substitute your wireless number in the free listings provided with your service (p. 61). 3) If non-phone number listing fees are high and many referrals come from phone directories, choose telephone messaging; if you plan alternate advertising for most referrals, forgo phone listings and choose paging or cellular messaging (p. 61). 4) If you choose a cellular phone for business and personal usage, to maintain role boundaries record a professional greeting and do not answer calls directly (pp. 61–62). 5) If you plan high call volume and/or more than one contact number, consider paging over cellular messaging (pp. 62–63).

Choosing a Messaging Service Company

If you choose a telephone line with voicemail for your messages, your choice of service may be limited to your local phone company. However, as more companies offer local service, you may be able to choose from more options. If so, and you want complimentary phone directory listings, be sure any company you are considering offers this benefit. Also make sure that you will receive all the voicemail features you want. If you plan to have paging service and a pager connected to your line, check that the telephone company offers this, too. Then compare rates for similar services so you can choose a company offering the most at the least expense to you.

When choosing paging and/or cellular service, you have a variety of options. A good place to start in your search is to ask what your colleagues, friends, and other people you know are using. Once you get some names, you can find them in the yellow pages or Internet and contact them to compare services and rates. If no one you know uses a paging service, you can go directly to the phone book or an Internet search for providers.

When comparing options, look for a large, nationwide company that has been in business for a long time. Although you may find some newer local or regional companies that offer even cheaper rates, these may not be as financially stable, offer as many features, or provide service in every state. As a result, they are more at risk of going out of business. If this happens, you will have to start all over and get new service, change your number, and put in the time and effort to notify everyone.

When I started using paging service, I did not look into these issues but immediately chose what my colleagues were using. Luckily it was a large, stable company and although it has changed names, it is still in business today. I have used the same service many years and now pay less monthly—about the cost of a lunch special—than when I started. Since it is a nationwide company, even if I moved out of state, I could keep the same service and rate, saving the cost and effort of changing systems.

Voicemail

Telephone and cellular phone service usually offer one voicemail package, so be sure that it includes the special features you want, such as call forwarding, and caller ID. In contrast, paging service typically offers many voicemail plans. If this will be your messaging service, get the best plan available, roughly comparable to standard phone service voicemail. Look for the following features: maximum recording time of greeting and incoming messages, the most calls saved, and the longest time kept. These premium features typically do not cost much more than other choices and are well worth the small additional fee.

When using voicemail as your answering system, every feature can affect the quality of your work. For example, when you have maximum time to record your greeting message, you can provide information without rushing. Since this will be your first and possibly only introduction to callers, it helps to have enough time to present your practice comfortably. When the recording capacity for messages is high, dropped calls will be prevented, important especially in time of crisis or with referral messages. If there is a limit to the number of saved messages and your calling volume is high, by checking messages regularly and deleting old ones, you can make sure to receive all calls before new ones replace them. For example, when using my paging system, I try to listen to messages as soon as my pager goes off, or every hour between sessions if I'm with clients. Also, when callers have plenty of time to leave messages, they will be able to complete their calls in peace without the frustration of being cut off too soon. Since many of your clients may be in acute distress, this will avoid adding to their grief.

Pager

If you choose a paging or telephone service with an additional paging option, you will need a pager to alert you of calls received. Typically you will need to buy one from the company you choose. If your telephone company does not sell them, you can find one in pager stores. Although there are many differently priced models, the most basic, called digital or numeric, is probably all you need. Since callers will be leaving voice messages on your voicemail, you only need the pager to alert you when a call is received. All pagers will do this through optional tones or vibrations.

Digital models also support an alternative option of numeric messaging, which I wouldn't recommend. In numeric messaging, a greeting message directs callers to enter their return number instead of leaving a voice message, and the digits are then displayed on your pager screen. The preferred voicemail option gives you much more information from calls, allowing you to screen out unwelcome advertisers or marketers before spending your valuable time returning calls. You can also distinguish between routine messages and client emergencies, returning calls as appropriate through whatever phone you choose. After buying the pager, you will also be charged a monthly fee to use the paging service. Depending on the company, this may be separate from or combined with voicemail fees.

You also have the option of a more expensive alphanumeric pager, which receives and displays numbers as well as text messages. Again, since your calls will be voice messages only, you would be paying for something you won't really need. You could even get a pricier 2-way pager, allowing you to also send and receive text messages through Internet email. With this option, not only is the pager much more expensive, but you will also need to pay much more for monthly service, again, something you don't really need. By buying the lowest priced digital model, you can keep expenses down and still receive the basic paging service you will use.

⊁ Replacement Plan

One more service option to consider is a replacement plan in case your pager is lost, stolen, or breaks. Some companies offer coverage for all three events and others may only replace a broken pager. Fees tend to range from one to four dollars extra per month. This replacement coverage is usually available for cellular phones as well. If you tend to lose or drop things it may be worth paying the extra monthly fee. However, if you are not prone to these slips, you can save by not paying more for this protection. Since pager and cell phone prices are so much lower these days compared to years ago, if you do have to buy a new one, it will be much easier to afford. Since starting paging service, I have never paid for this coverage, and so far I haven't lost or broken my pager. As a result, the savings benefit has been more than enough to pay for many new pagers.

Changing Your Messaging System

If you currently have a secretary, answering service, or another phone message system, an opportune time to switch to a lower cost messaging option is when you change office locations or practice arrangements. I did this when leaving the large group practice I described earlier, with daytime secretarial service and an after-hours answering system. In moving to a smaller expense-sharing group, I transitioned to the individual paging service my colleagues were using. Although it took time and effort to set this up and notify everyone of the phone number change, once it was done, the monthly savings and benefits quickly compensated for the task. Even if you are not planning a move, you could still change messaging systems to receive the same benefits.

Issue	Recommendation
Choosing and changing your messaging system.	1) To ensure uninterrupted messaging service, select a large, nationwide company that has been in business for a long time (p. 64). 2) To enhance the quality of your work, choose voicemail with the features you want, offering the longest time to record and save the most messages (pp. 64–65). 3) For cost-effective quality paging, buy a basic pager; for maximum information and screening of calls use voicemail versus numeric messaging (pp. 65–66). 4) If you frequently drop or lose your pager/cellular phone, consider monthly replacement coverage; if you are not prone to these slips, save by skipping this option (p. 66). 5) To switch from secretarial/answering service to a low cost messaging system, a convenient time is when you change office locations or practice arrangements (p. 66).

Communications System Tips

Various practices can help you increase savings and service in your communication system. They involve paging and cellular work numbers, service plans, and caller ID blocking.

Paging and Cellular Work Numbers

If you choose a paging or cellular messaging system, make sure your number has an area code and prefix as central to your practice location as possible. Assuming you will use this as your public work number, it will be the one that clients, colleagues, insurance companies, and anyone else will call to reach you. Whereas telephone companies automatically assign numbers directly reflecting physical locations, paging and cellular companies may not. By having a number matching your location, you offer a convenient, local access number for callers. Plus, if the area code changes where you are practicing, your number will also reflect that change. Although this is unlikely, it can happen when new area codes are added or current ones shift boundaries due to population increases.

To ensure a central number, when signing up for service, ask the agent for a number as close to your office address as possible. Verify that the number matches the same area code of the city and, if possible, specific area of the city in which you are practicing. Sometimes numbers will be automatically assigned after signing up for service; if so, check the number as soon as you get it to be sure it reflects your office location.

Service Plans

Save on your communication system by choosing a service plan that closely matches what you will use. If you don't know your usage, determine this by monitoring your call volume over a period of time (e.g., two months) to determine what you typically need. This may not be relevant for paging service, which generally charges a flat service rate, but it is important in telephone and cellular phone service for which various plans are available based on call volume. You can find current service plan rates by calling customer service or searching company websites.

After choosing a service plan, check periodically (every six months or year) for cheaper plans offering the same or better service. Companies are constantly competing with each other to attract new customers; therefore, they are continually generating new service plans and better rates, although no one will call to tell you. This applies to paging and Internet service as well. Watch for new trends, like bundling multiple services (e.g., local, long distance calls, cellular phone, Internet) together for a cheaper rate, where, depending on your usage, you might be able to save significantly.

When writing this chapter, I called my telephone, paging, cellular, and Internet companies and asked for better rates. The telephone and cellular agents offered new plans with more monthly minutes at no extra cost, so I changed to these better options right away. The paging service reduced my monthly fee by 20 percent, for the same service I had before. Most notably, my monthly Internet service fee, offering unlimited usage, was lowered by 60 percent. All these savings came from simple inquiry calls; I just asked if there were any cheaper plans or rates for the service I was using. Granted, it had been more than a year since I had called about Internet and paging rates, and I am a long-standing customer with all businesses except the telephone company. However, even if you don't get all fees reduced when you call, you are likely to get some discounts. And if you don't periodically ask, you can be sure your rates will never change.

Caller ID Blocking

When making calls from phones you want to keep private, order complete caller ID blocking to protect your numbers, especially your home phone. There is typically no cost to do this and it only requires one phone call. Many people have caller ID and if you do not block your number, anyone using this feature can obtain it when you call them. Although most people would not violate your privacy by calling your number identified in this way, some clients could mistakenly call thinking it is your office phone. Others, especially those with more severe illnesses and/or poor boundaries, could call at all hours during the day or night.

I was reminded of this after purchasing a cellular phone to make personal and professional calls, but not ordering caller ID blocking. Weeks went by with no indication that anyone could identify my number until a very observant client pointed out that my private number showed up on his caller ID. I was lucky because he shared this out of concern for my privacy; if another client had reacted differently there could have been unwanted calls and a boundary issue to address in requesting not to call the number. Once advised, I immediately called the cellular company and ordered complete blocking. Even if the risk of someone abusing your confidential numbers may be small, it only takes one client to create a sense of violated privacy and anxiety in receiving future calls.

Sometimes you may call someone who does not accept blocked calls; in these cases you need to use another phone to make these calls. Office, cellular, or public pay phones are some options. Whatever you do, make sure to never unblock your most private number, usually your home line.

Note that any time you call a toll-free number your number will automatically show even if you have caller ID blocking. Before calling one of these numbers, consider who you are calling, how important confidentiality is, and choose a phone accordingly. For instance, whenever I call clients at their toll-free work numbers, I always use the office or cell phone, even when calling from home. Although a call from home would cost nothing, it is worth paying for a cell phone call to preserve my home privacy. On the other hand, when calling insurance companies, I routinely call from home. Calls can get lengthy when I'm placed on hold, and the savings from the high call volume outweighs the privacy concern, especially because I am not directly contacting clients.

When talking with anyone during an unblocked return call, emphasize the correct public work number at which to reach you in the future. For example, if you make unblocked calls from an office fax line, explain that you are calling from a dedicated fax line and remind people to always call your work number to reach you. When calling from a cellular phone, do not share that you are using a cell phone; instead, simply give the directive to call your public work number for future calls. This reduces the risk of boundary issues arising from knowledge that you carry a cell phone. Keeping your choice of a cellular or pager messaging system private is a good habit to have, helping to reduce unnecessary client calls and unhealthy dependencies.

Issue	Recommendation
Increasing savings and service in your communications system.	1) For convenient access for nearby callers, make sure your cellular/paging contact number is as central to your office as possible (pp. 67–68). 2) For the most savings, choose a service plan matching only what you need, monitoring your calling volume to determine average usage (p. 68). 3) For the best service and lowest rates, periodically call (e.g. six months to one year) and ask for better deals (p. 68). 4) To protect your personal privacy, order caller ID blocking on any phones you want to keep confidential (p. 69). 5) To prevent dropped calls and boundary problems, during unblocked return calls, state the correct public work number at which to reach you in the future, keeping your usage of a cellular or paging messaging system private (pp. 69–70).

PART II
Simplifying Daily Procedures

CHAPTER FOUR

Streamlining for the First Appointment

The process of arranging for initial appointments is crucial to every private practice. By following the steps detailed in this chapter, you can complete this process quickly and comprehensively, attending to clients' needs as well as your own. You will learn how to protect client privacy when returning calls, preventing draining conflicts with others who answer your calls instead. These tips will help you quickly screen clients for compatibility, checking for hidden agendas that don't match your services. You will discover how to discuss fee and insurance issues in advance to ensure complete and prompt payment for services. Further steps will guide you in scheduling, giving directions, and providing instructions unique to your practice, helping clients to follow through with your services and arrive to appointments on time.

Screening and Scheduling Clients Yourself

One benefit of scheduling clients yourself, as opposed to having a staff person do it, is that you can establish a personal connection right away, helping people feel comfortable making an appointment with you and following through with treatment. You also retain complete control over the quality of services they receive. Additionally, by retaining the income you would have paid someone else to set appointments, you gain more flexibility in deciding how many clients to see. For example, if you want to reduce therapy hours to lower daily stress or pursue another professional activity, you can more easily afford to do this than if you are paying for office staff to handle scheduling.

For these reasons and more, I personally prefer to be my own office manager. I also like varying direct therapy and business tasks; this balance helps preserve energy and adds longevity to my practice. I suspect if I had a secretary I would be constantly double-checking things anyway, duplicating services and wasting time and money. Whether your preference is like mine, or you'd rather hire someone else, there are steps you can take that benefit everyone and, in turn, increase the quality of your work.

Confidentiality

One of the first issues to consider in setting initial appointments is confidentiality. When you return calls to prospective clients, you may not reach them right away; spouses, roommates, parents, employers, etc. could answer the phone. Although their relationship with your client could be kind and supportive, they could also be filled with conflicts and perhaps even be the main trigger for them to seek help. Information you share could make the situation worse, compromising your client's well-being and damaging therapy before it even gets started. By remaining discreet during attempts to speak with new clients, you can safeguard privacy and avoid adding to their distress, preserving the therapeutic alliance and process from the beginning. Demonstrating this kind of care may also increase the chance that they will choose you as their therapist.

I was reminded just how important confidentiality is when calling a prospective client named Tony back the first time. Tony was a busy professional in sales and had left a message inquiring about my services, including his office and home numbers. After leaving a voicemail message at his work number, I called his home and was immediately greeted by a woman who shared that he was not there but she would be happy to take a message. She also asked what the call was regarding. Instead of telling her or leaving a message, I simply offered that I was returning Tony's call and would call his office instead.

After reaching Tony, I was relieved that I had not shared anything. It turned out that when he left his message, he included his home number by mistake and was confidentially calling for treatment for a sexual addiction. His wife knew nothing about his problem and plan for treatment, and he was not ready to tell her anything at the time. If I had innocently shared the nature of my call, privacy would have been destroyed, distress would peak, and Tony would be unlikely to choose my services, or more importantly, anyone else's. This example shows that you can never be sure what's going on in prospective clients' lives, why they want to see you, what their relationships are like, what they are comfortable sharing, and most importantly, what they want to keep private.

Steps to Ensure Confidentiality

A first step you can take to preserve confidentiality is to respond to clients' inquiry calls as soon as possible. The sooner you call back, the more chance you have of reaching them directly versus dealing with someone else, bypassing the privacy problem from the beginning. By using a communications system described in Chapter 3, you can ensure quick return calls. However, there will always be times you don't immediately reach clients and in these situations you can proceed with the following steps.

When someone answers your call, preserve confidentiality by asking for the client by name as opposed to automatically assuming the person you are talking with is the client (e.g., "Is Mary Rogers there?"). If the client is home but the person answering asks you to identify yourself before turning over the phone, you can say your name without your title ("This is Ann Smith"). Here you continue to honor confidentiality by not disclosing your professional identity or relationship to the client. If the person still asks, "What is this regarding?," you can say, "I am returning her call." Sometimes people persist and in these cases you can say, "I'm returning her call so I'm not sure."

Though most people do not go this far in grilling you, it is important to know before the call starts how you will handle these questions while honoring privacy. As my earlier experience shows, you never know who is on the other end of the phone and what that person's relationship is to the client. If you unknowingly disclose information that the prospective client wanted to be kept private, the therapy and your client could already be harmed before the first session, especially if treatment was planned in secret.

Often people will leave return contact numbers along with directives to call during certain times, increasing your chances of directly reaching them. However, if they are not available when you call back and you get an answering machine or another person, you can preserve privacy by leaving your name and phone number without your title or any reference to therapy. You can do the same when calling clients back at work. Sometimes receptionists may ask what company you are calling from and in these cases you can say, simply, "My office." When using business as opposed to mental health terms as identifiers, you safeguard confidentiality by not arousing curiosity about your services. You may also be asked by a receptionist what the call is regarding, and again you can say, "I am returning his/her call" or "He/She will know what this call is in reference to."

My colleague Megan's experience shows just how useful these initial steps can be. She returned a new client inquiry call at her work, and when a woman answered, she asked to speak with Sue. Although this woman was not Sue, she was very friendly and offered to take a message. Megan left her name and number, but the woman further asked why she was calling and offered to help out in any way. Megan kept her response short, saying she was returning a call. Later, after talking with Sue, she found out that Sue was filing a worker's compensation claim due to job stress. The major trigger of Sue's distress came from dealing with her supervisor, the same woman who answered Megan's call and was so persistent in requests for information. As Megan's careful approach demonstrates, by keeping your messages short and free of descriptive information, you can maintain privacy and avoid adding to problems before therapy begins.

Issue	Recommendation
Securing confidentiality when contacting prospective clients for initial apppointments.	1) To enhance client comfort, ensure follow-through with treatment, quality service, and gain financial flexibility, schedule your own client appointments (pp. 73–74). 2) To preserve confidentiality, return inquiry calls as quickly as possible, ask for the client by name, and do not disclose your professional identity, your relationship to the client, or the nature of the call (pp. 74–75). 3) To ensure privacy when leaving messages for potential clients, leave only your name and phone number without your title or any reference to therapy; if asked why you are calling say "I am returning his/her call" (pp. 75–76).

Screen for Compatibility

Once you directly reach clients, find out if your services are a good match for their needs. By addressing this issue right away, you can save everyone the time, work, and money that would have been spent setting up the appointment only to discover later that the client needs to go somewhere else.

To start, introduce yourself: "Hello, this is Dr. Jim Jackson. I am returning your phone call. How can I help you?" This reminds clients who you are and that you are responding to their request. Often they will begin by asking for an appointment and/or inquire about your rates. Before arranging a time or discussing payment, first raise questions to determine compatibility.

Ask, "Can you tell me briefly what brings you to talk with me?" Clients' answers will help you identify incompatible referrals immediately—for example, a child referral when you see only adults, a request for group therapy when you do not have a group. It may be tempting to respond to therapy requests by adjusting your services to ensure referrals and fill client spots, but in the long run you will find this leads to more problems than benefits, especially if you are stretching well beyond your practice comfort zone.

If you are getting started in practice you may not know exactly where to draw the line with certain referrals. By carefully observing your performance, comfort level, and preference as you work with various clients, you can refine your boundaries and gain clarity about which new prospects should be referred to providers outside your scope of practice. A clear policy on this matter will help clients connect to the best resources for their needs while preserving your well-being and practice longevity at the same time. When refining your practice limits, it is helpful to research who offers the services you do not, then you will have immediate referrals to offer clients and be able to assist your colleagues in increasing their clientele. By directing prospective clients to share your name as the referring party, your fellow clinicians will also be more likely to think of you when they have referrals, and reciprocate by sending clients your way.

When starting out in practice I went through this process after accepting couples and family therapy cases, quickly realizing I was working beyond my preference and comfort level. Although I had some training in these modalities, I did not enjoy the work and felt my skills and interests were better suited to individual therapy. After these experiences, I decided to limit my practice to individual therapy only. When people called requesting couples and family therapy, I said, "Unfortunately I do not provide couples/family therapy, but if you would like referrals to other therapists who do, I can give you some names and numbers." For those who requested referrals I asked, "When you call Ms. Perez, be sure to tell her I sent you her way, so she will know how you found her." I discovered that clients were usually grateful to receive personal referrals, and therapists to whom I had referred clients were likely to refer individual clients back to me.

When referring people elsewhere, you can also encourage them to call back if they ever need your services in the future. For example, when I refer people to couples therapists I say, "Also, if you or anyone else you know would like individual therapy in the future, feel free to call me back at any time." Such call-backs can happen more often than you may think, especially as people get started in therapy and discover additional services they or their loved ones need.

For instance, after referring a woman who asked for marital therapy to resolve conflicts with her husband, she called back a few weeks later requesting individual therapy. With the help of marital intervention they were getting along better, and she was realizing her low self-esteem, poor body image, and lack of assertiveness had been contributing to the conflicts. With her husband's support, she was now ready to work on these issues individually. Another woman who I referred to couples therapy called back two weeks later requesting individual therapy after her husband refused to enter therapy with her. She was tired of trying to engage him in counseling and wanted help to sort out her own feelings. These are just some of the many scenarios that can lead people back to you. You never know when clients' needs may change, and when you directly encourage them to call, even when referring them elsewhere, they will likely think of you and feel comfortable calling in the future when needing the services you do offer.

Hidden Agendas

Sometimes you may find that people initially state one reason for seeking therapy over the phone and then later in person reveal an entirely different request outside your realm of practice. When you know your practice limits, you can directly ask clients whether they expect certain services you do not offer, and if so, direct them to someone who does. The exact questions to ask will depend on your specific practice boundaries, and you may need time to develop and refine them as you gain experience with typical requests not matching your services.

ADDITIONAL EXAMPLES OF HIDDEN AGENDAS TO UNCOVER BEFORE INITIAL APPOINTMENTS	
Presenting Agendas	**Hidden Agendas**
• Work-related stress	• Desires letters or court appearances for lawsuits (e.g., sexual harassment, job discrimination, change in job duties).
• Family and child issues	• Desires letters of support to courts/agencies for divorce, change of teacher or schools for child, adoption.
• Economic troubles	• Wants payment deferred.
• Seeking specific therapy technique	• Wants technique used in a way you do not practice (e.g., hypnosis to recover memories of abuse).

One example comes from a professional acquaintance of mine named Ann, who primarily works with families and children. When first starting in practice, she began to notice a frustrating trend. Parents would seek her services stating that they wanted help for themselves and their children coping with the stress of impending divorce. When she met them in person, they added that they were in a heated battle for the children and wanted a custody evaluation for the courts. Since Ann did not specialize in this service, she had to inform them in session of her limits and refer them to someone else, taking much time, effort, and adding to everyone's distress. Now she specifically asks parents who are divorcing the following over the phone, "Do you want me to perform a custody evaluation for the courts?," and if they do, she explains her limits and refers them right away to colleagues who do provide this service.

Other requests I have encountered include people seeking disability evaluations, legal reports and involvement in various court matters, requesting payment to be deferred, and wanting therapy techniques I do not provide. Before learning to ask questions to identify these hidden agendas right away, I had to inform clients sometimes well into therapy that I could not fulfill their requests as they were outside my practice parameters.

For example, one new client shared over the phone that she wanted help to reduce job stress. She was feeling anxious, depressed, and overwhelmed by her job requirements at the phone company. She was also stressed out dealing with the demands of her family, husband, and children. Her issues sounded like a good match with my services so we proceeded in scheduling her first session, which went very well until the last five minutes when she pulled out some forms from her purse, sharing that the physician who referred her said I could evaluate her for disability and complete the required paperwork. In addition, she stated that she needed the paperwork completed that day so she could receive payment for time off work. My stress level peaked as I explained that although I could offer therapy for her job stress, I did not provide disability evaluations, and I described the reasons why. I then had to refer her to someone who provided this service, adding to her frustration and delaying her session until this was resolved. Now if someone calls for help with job stress, I immediately ask over the phone, "Are you considering taking leave from work due to stress?" and "Are you looking for someone to evaluate you for disability leave from work?" If so, I share my limits and immediately refer them to others who offer this service.

Your practice parameters may be very different; perhaps you do custody or disability evaluations. Or, your specialty may be forensic work and you are comfortable working with legal matters. By identifying what you do and don't do, you can continually refine the questions you ask potential clients during inquiry calls, building a clientele whose needs match what you offer and referring others to more compatible services.

Before ending or continuing calls, ask, "I'm curious, how did you receive my name?" By monitoring where referrals are coming from, you can market to your most reliable referral sources when needed and discontinue any strategies that aren't working. For example, say you have placed three expensive ads in the local newspaper but no one has responded; instead, most of your clients are finding you through no-cost insurance lists. With this knowledge you can discontinue the advertisements, saving the time and cost of this fruitless endeavor.

Practice Description

After confirming that you offer what callers want, share a brief description of your background and current practice, covering the following areas:

ISSUES TO COVER IN YOUR PRACTICE DESCRIPTION	
• Education and licensure	• Session length
• Places you have worked	• Specialties
• Private practice experience	• Therapy approach
	• Unique training

This description takes just a minute or two to share and will also highlight features to help you stand out as a therapist. Clients almost always will appreciate the information offered; sometimes they will ask for this on their own, but many will not, simply because it slips their mind or they do not know what questions to ask.

This information will help clients better understand the nature and value of your services, as well as your individual style and approach. With this knowledge, they are also more likely to feel comfortable starting therapy with you. As many clients may find you in directories and impersonal listings, by personally offering a description of your background and work, chances are they will choose you more often over someone they know nothing about.

One sample description my former office mate used is as follows: "I am a licensed marriage and family therapist and have worked for the past few years in a community clinic, a hospital, and my current private practice. I provide individual, family, and couples therapy for a range of issues, and my sessions are forty-five minutes long. In my approach, I first offer coping strategies to help clients feel better quickly. Then, I assist people in identifying destructive patterns they may be repeating, helping them to change to newer, healthier habits and roles in relationships. I offer a special family therapy technique using audio/video feedback I find to be very useful in helping people. If you would like to know more about this I would be happy to tell you."

example...

Your own practice description will likely be different, reflecting your unique background, orientation, and specialties. Maybe you have psychoanalytic training or work with children with learning disorders. Perhaps you have a substance abuse specialty or a particular marital therapy approach. By highlighting your strengths and interests, you will attract clients wanting your services. Throughout your practice life periodically review and update any features that change. By keeping your description up to date, you can facilitate the best match between what you currently offer and what potential clients are looking for at that time. Although during inquiry calls it's best if your description is brief, you can also provide a more comprehensive summary in writing to clients when they arrive for a first appointment.

Issue	Recommendation
Screening prospective clients for compatibility before setting initial appointments.	1) To screen for compatibility, ask clients to describe the services they want, immediately referring those whose requests do not match what you offer (pp. 77–78). 2) To increase future referrals, ask clients to tell the referred-to therapists that you sent them; encourage clients and others they know to call if they need future services you provide (p. 78). 3) To save time, money, and unneeded stress, probe for hidden agendas by directly asking clients if they want specific services you do not offer (e.g., custody evaluation), referring those with incompatible expectations (pp. 78–80). 4) To monitor referrals and adjust your marketing efforts, ask clients how they got your name (p. 80). 5) To help clients understand the nature and value of your services, briefly describe your background and current practice (pp. 80–81). 6) To facilitate the best match between client requests and your services, periodically update your practice description, and provide a comprehensive written summary in the first session (pp. 81–82).

Payment

Once you determine compatibility you can say something like, "Because the issues you are describing are ones that I deal with often, I think we would be a good match in working together." People can easily go on at length telling you about their problems, not realizing how much time they are taking. This reassurance helps cue them to continue the process of setting an appointment. The next important issue to discuss is payment, where you can confirm the method and your rates.

Self Pay

If you do not work with insurance and/or for clients not using insurance benefits for services, continue with, "Are you planning to pay for services yourself?" If so, "Let me tell you about my rates. My fee for a _____ minute session is _____ dollars". Some clients will be fine with this and you can proceed with, "I accept cash or check for the amount due at each session. Which of these methods are you planning to use for payments?" By confirming the exact amount and how they will pay, clients will be fully informed before coming to their first session, reducing the chances of misunderstandings and failure to pay once they arrive at your office.

If you accept credit cards, you can also include this payment option. Although I do not, my colleague, Bill, does; he finds it to be well worth the extra processing fees. He obtains credit card billing information during initial calls and also informs clients of his cancellation policy. In addition to charging for attended sessions, if clients do not show, he bills their credit card for the amount due, ensuring payment for missed visits. If you want to learn more about becoming a credit card merchant, your local bank is a good place to start. Other large discount stores (e.g., Costco) or professional organizations (e.g., American Psychological Association) may also offer these services.

Credit cards?

Some prospective clients may express financial difficulty in paying your fee, and if so, you can either refer them to other, lower cost services or consider offering a reduced rate. Whatever your fees, it's always helpful to have two or more low and/or no cost referral options available. Some people will not be able to afford your services and for them you will have resources to offer within their means; "You can also call a clinic called Therapy Services Are Us. They have a sliding fee scale and a variety of therapists available. Their number is (phone number). Even if they do not work out you can ask them for other referrals too. If you want to see a private therapist you may also try (therapist name) at (phone number). I'm not sure how low her sliding scale goes but you can call and ask if you want."

Sliding Fee Scale

When deciding whether to offer a sliding fee scale, do not view it as a routine option for clients. Think of it instead as an exception to offer clients in financial distress who cannot afford your usual rates. Keep in mind that lowering clients' payments when they are using insurance benefits is considered fraudulent by third party payers because your collected fee is lower than your billed fee to insurance. One way to prevent this problem is to not use a sliding fee scale for insured clients. For anyone else that you do see at a lower rate, document your reasons in detail. Then, if any problems arise, you will be able to show in writing the rationale you used to justify your fee in that individual case.

In my practice, I do have a sliding fee scale but I use it rarely. A majority of my clientele uses insurance benefits to pay for services and they almost always can afford their payment responsibility. The occasional times I do offer a reduced fee happen when self-pay clients are unable to afford standard rates. Since my practice is in a city with a large lower- and middle-class population, this issue does arise at times. When these financially distressed clients have presenting issues matching my specialties, and I am available to take them on as clients, I turn to the back-up sliding fee option.

You may not want to offer a sliding scale or be uncomfortable offering reduced fees. Whatever your preference, it is important to have a firm policy established before talking to prospective clients so you know what you will and will not offer. If you decide to have a sliding scale, be sure to set your fee range and feel comfortable with both ends before talking with prospective clients. You want to feel worth your top fee but not resentful of your lowest rate. When setting your bottom fee, a financially safe approach is to select a fee that will cover your expenses and earn an acceptable income even if all your clients paid this rate.

One factor you can consider in setting a sliding fee scale is your experience, with higher fees commensurate with more years in practice. For example, over the years my fee range has narrowed: when first in practice I offered a bottom rate that was a 40 percent discount from my standard fee. Now, after gaining more experience and skills, the most I reduce fees is 20 percent. In your own practice, it's helpful to review your rates periodically and adjust them to reflect your experience, skills, and comfort level. This includes raising your highest as well as your lowest fee. These adjustments will prevent you from selling yourself short over time, preserve your income and job satisfaction, and, in turn, enhance your effectiveness at delivering services.

When presenting a sliding fee scale, make sure the method you choose is comfortable for you and does not harm the delicate client-therapist relationship you are already developing. The method that I prefer is to first predetermine the lowest rate you could offer clients while still honoring your financial needs and professional self-worth. Then, when offering a reduced fee you can say, "I do offer a sliding fee schedule starting at the standard rate of _____ dollars to my lowest fee of _____ dollars. I would be happy to offer you the lowest fee to give you a break financially." Clients are almost always appreciative of this offer and it saves the stress of negotiating your service fee. Since you have already determined the lowest financially and professionally viable rate, you ensure adequate compensation to meet your bottom line and avoid selling yourself too short.

Issue	Recommendation
Discussing fees, payment, and sliding scales with prospective self-pay clients.	1) To inform self-pay clients and ensure compensation at the time of service, share your exact fee and confirm their method of payment (pp. 82–83). 2) To provide affordable services to clients who cannot pay your fee, give them two or more low/no cost referral options, or offer a reduced fee (p. 83). 3) When using a sliding fee scale, offer it as an exception only for clients in severe financial distress who cannot afford your rate, documenting the reasons in detail that justify lowering your fee (pp. 83–84). 4) To set a fee range that is comfortable and financially safe for you, select a bottom rate that will yield an acceptable income if all your clients paid that rate; choose a top rate commensurate with your experience, periodically reviewing and adjusting your range (p. 84). 5) To protect the delicate client-therapist relationship, avoid stressful negotiations and offer instead your lowest professionally viable rate to financially disadvantaged clients (pp. 84–85).

Insurance Check

If you do accept insurance, ask clients to provide identifying information for their policies so you can later call their insurance carriers to thoroughly check benefits before their first appointments. It may seem like a lot of work to investigate benefits before even seeing clients, but it can be invaluable in saving everyone's money and frustration later. The risk in not checking is that you may believe there is insurance coverage and then later after you have seen clients four or five times, you could be denied payment for your services (it's usually at least a month turnaround from first paper billing to payment). You are then stuck with the unpleasant task of telling clients that not only did their insurance deny services, but also they now have a large and unexpected bill. They could become angry and stop therapy, leaving you with unpaid services and little chance of recouping your losses. Clients could also suffer therapeutically if they associate the work done with the negative experience of the insurance disaster. Their distress could even prevent them from seeking therapy in the future. If they do, they may begin with a negative expectation, detracting from the gains they could be making. If this happens, you or the new therapist will assume the added task of helping them recover from this negative experience before even resuming the previous therapy work.

My colleague, Jim, quickly realized the importance of checking insurance benefits when he was first starting in practice. He was eager to build his clientele and was pleased to accept a new referral, assuming that insurance would cover the new client's visits. Therefore, he did not ask for benefit details ahead of time or call the insurance company to verify coverage. Meanwhile, he successfully worked with this client, finishing in ten sessions. Since he did not bill frequently for services, by the time the insurance company responded his client was long gone. To his shock, the insurance denied payment for all his sessions, stating that he needed precertification in order for his services to be covered. Although he then billed his client for the outstanding total, he never heard back or received any payment. To this day, he now confirms benefits for every insured client, remembering in vivid detail the hard lesson he learned upon opening that fateful letter from the insurance company.

As more and more insurance shifts to managed care and preferred provider plans, the question of whether your services are covered becomes even more crucial. In Jim's example, he assumed his client's insurance did not require case management. In fact, in previous years it did not, but that year the rules were changed to require preauthorization. As rules and benefits continue to change more frequently, verifying current coverage is increasingly critical to preventing problems like Jim encountered.

Many clients may not check on benefits themselves before calling you, especially if they have been directly referred from physicians' offices or friends and family. Even those who do may get your name from outdated or inaccurate insurance lists. Clients you have seen in the past may reinitiate therapy and it's important to do the same insurance check with them again, as their benefits may have changed since you last saw them.

Even though the services I offered were not covered at all by a particular insurance company, I was once listed for an entire year as a psychiatrist in their directory. This insurance paid only for medication visits; it did not cover psychotherapy services. If I hadn't checked benefits before initial sessions and referred these clients to psychiatrists, they could have become very upset in my office after learning I did not provide medications, not to mention that the insurer would have denied all my billed charges for these appointments.

Check Benefits Yourself

It may be tempting to rely on clients to do their own benefit check, saving you the time and hassle of performing this less-than-desirable task. However, you run the risk of clients not knowing what to ask and receiving incorrect or misleading information. It's a challenge to deal with the rules and details of mental health benefits even if you are familiar with the errors that can occur. To expect that clients will be able to navigate these frequently dysfunctional systems puts them and you at risk of assuming certain benefits and later finding out that services were not covered or paid at a much lower rate than expected.

Even when clients confidently tell you their payment responsibility, they may be incorrectly quoting co-pays for general medical visits, often lower than psychotherapy fees. These medical co-pays are usually printed on insurance cards that clients may read and assume apply for all their health services, including mental health.

You can start by advising clients in the following manner: "Since you are planning to use insurance benefits to pay for services, you are responsible for knowing what your plan covers and for paying any fees that insurance does not pay. To help you out with this, as a courtesy to prospective new clients, I provide the service of verifying insurance benefits. I am happy to do this for you." Clients are almost always pleased and appreciative that you would go to the trouble to double check their benefits. By taking this active, supportive step to facilitate treatment, you will strengthen rapport, reduce your clients' distress, and protect yourself financially.

Staying on Track with Insurance Questions

As you continue with insurance questions during your initial conversation with prospective clients, and anytime during the phone call, you may find that clients redirect their answers to focus on their presenting problems. To complete your protocol efficiently while preserving rapport, you can say, "Those are very important issues and I look forward to talking about them in our first session. If you would like to write them down so you don't forget, please bring in your notes so we can refer to them when you come in." Many times this will be enough to cue people to move on; however, if not, you can add, "I have another appointment (obligation, commitment) starting soon, so I just have a couple minutes left for us to finish setting up our first meeting. We'll need to move on but please remember to bring these important issues to our session."

To proceed, follow this protocol to find out what clients know about their insurance coverage:

ASKING CLIENTS WHAT THEY KNOW ABOUT THEIR INSURANCE COVERAGE

1) Are you planning to use any insurance benefits for these services?
2) What is the name of your insurance company?
3) Did you call your insurance company to ask for a therapist referral?
4) Did you get an authorization to see me?
5) What is your authorization number?
6) How many visits were authorized?
7) What is your co-payment for each visit?
8) Does your insurance plan have a deductible?
9) How much is it?

For insurance plans you are certain you don't accept, you can inform clients immediately, saving everyone the time and effort that would have been spent setting up a first appointment and later finding out they can't use their benefits to pay you. However, if you are at all uncertain about clients' coverage, continue with all of the questions. Write down all the answers so later you can compare them to what you are told when you call the insurance provider to directly verify benefits.

ENSURING ACCURATE INFORMATION. People may give you the name of their insurance thinking that it covers their entire healthcare (e.g., Blue Shield or Prudential) when instead, a different insurance company, usually managed care, handles mental health benefits separately. If clients have a specific authorization, they are typically covered through a managed care plan. Once you are familiar with different companies' authorization protocols, it is easier to identify them when clients answer these questions. With some insurance, customer service agents will first offer referrals, directing clients to call back for certification once they choose a therapist and set an appointment. Other plans with unrestricted benefits will not require authorization or ongoing case management.

Often clients have no idea whether their insurance covers therapy and may assume that since they are covered for medical treatment, they are also covered for mental health services. They may not have called their insurance provider and probably do not know that for some plans there is a required authorization and they must see an in-network therapist in order to use their benefits. This may be their first time to engage in therapy services and the last thing they may be thinking about is insurance coverage. Most likely they are probably focused on the issues for which they are seeking therapy.

ASKING CLIENTS FOR IDENTIFYING INFORMATION ON THEIR INSURANCE CARDS

1) Do you have your insurance card available?
2) Is this insurance in your name or someone else's (husband, wife, father, mother)?
3) Can you spell the name for me?
4) (If the insured is not the client) Can you also spell your full name for me?
5) What is (the insured's) ID number, often it is the social security number on the card.
6) What is (the insured's) birth date?
7) (If the insured is not the client) What is your birth date?
8) What is the group number?
9) What is the employer's name?
10) What is the phone number of the insurance company?
11) If you look on the front or back of your insurance card, does it say something like this: For mental health call (800) 000-0000?
12) Can you please read what it says?
13) (If clients read only a phone number ask) Is there a name or initials next to the number (e.g., Managed Health Network or MHN)?
14) Can you please read what it says?
15) Are you covered by a second insurance, too? If yes, go back to question 1 and repeat the protocol for the second insurance carrier. Note: Married clients and minors often have more than one insurance plan.

Even if they have been aware of insurance details in the past, their current level of anxiety or depression or other symptoms may preclude them from remembering or taking steps to verify coverage on their own.

INSURANCE IDENTIFIERS. To proceed in obtaining accurate information to verify clients' benefits, ask clients to refer to their insurance card to help you answer the questions on page 89. Clients usually have their insurance card nearby, in their purse or wallet, and can take it out and read it as you talk on the phone.

Scheduling the First Session

Once you receive insurance information from clients, you can proceed in scheduling the first session. This allows you to complete referrals right away when clients are available and motivated, and you still have time to call and verify coverage well before the session. Continue with, "I will call your insurance company and if the benefits are any different from what we discussed, I'll call before our first appointment to let you know. Unless you hear differently from me your payment for the first session will be ____ dollars. Either cash or check will be fine." By stating the exact fee you prevent incorrect assumptions and facilitate payment at the first session.

If you don't yet know the benefits or correct co-pay, you can say, "I will call your insurance company and then call you back to tell you your benefits and payment. You can bring either cash or a check to your session." Then, call the insurance provider and client back as soon as possible to fully inform them of their payment responsibility. If they decide not to engage your services, you can refer them elsewhere and still have enough time to offer the appointment to another referral.

You can add, "If you would like to go ahead yourself and doublecheck the benefits that would be fine, too, then we can compare notes on what each of us was told." Usually clients are more than happy to leave it to you to check on this, but you are offering them control in checking for themselves, and this may be especially important for clients with initial trust and autonomy concerns.

For clients with managed care who have not yet completed initial certifications you can say, "Please call your insurance company back right away to tell them our first appointment time and complete the authorization. Then please call me back with the certification number, the number of visits, and your co-pay." When clients complete this task you are assured of insurance payments for services.

Full Fee versus Co-Pay

You may be wondering why clients are directed to bring only their co-payments to visits. Perhaps you know colleagues who collect full fees at every session, even for clients with insurance. Therapists who do this typically give clients a statement of services provided at each session—called a super bill—directing them to bill insurance on their own for reimbursement. If you see clients with unrestricted insurance who can afford full payments, do their own billing, and wait for reimbursement, you may prefer this approach.

However, this plan will not work for clients with managed care or other insurance for which you sign a contract as a preferred provider. Contracts usually prohibit you from collecting more than co-pays from clients, even if you will later reimburse them. They often require billing on special claim forms with authorization numbers and other identifiers not known to the client. Many insurance plans will only pay bills submitted by the provider of service and deny payments if any required billing details are incorrect. Additionally, your contracted rates are usually lower than your customary fees. If you charge clients your full fee up front, you run the risk of overcharging with negative ethical, legal, and therapeutic consequences. For these reasons, your best approach is to calculate expected payments from both insurance companies and clients, and collect only the clients' portion due at each session.

Issue	Recommendation
Confirming insurance coverage, initial certifications, and client fees.	1) To accommodate available and motivated clients, proceed to schedule sessions, sharing exact fees due if known; immediately call insurance for coverage and if needed, call clients back with correct benefit and payment information (p. 90). 2) To assure insurance payment for services, ask clients to complete initial authorizations when needed and call you back with the details (pp. 90–91). 3) To prevent overcharging clients and insurance payment denials, calculate expected payments from insurance providers and clients, collecting only client portions due at each session (p. 91).

Choosing an Appointment Time

After addressing payment and insurance issues, you can continue by asking, "Would you like to go ahead and set a time for our first appointment?" If yes, "Is your schedule fairly flexible?" If you find out clients' availability first you have more discretion to choose a matching time that is open in your schedule. In contrast, if you first ask clients when they would like to come, they may request peak times when they could be seen at other times, thereby crowding out other prospective clients with a more limited schedule.

Clients may respond by saying they can only see you on certain days or times when you do not work (e.g., Friday evening or Saturday). If so, it is helpful to tell them right away that you have a set schedule, including times that are already booked: "I have client appointments on Mondays and Tuesdays with a range of times from morning to evening, but the early morning and late afternoon and evening times are very popular and often spoken for already." Before talking with prospective clients, check your schedule for the next two or three weeks so you will know what appointments you can offer. For example, "I do have an opening next Tuesday at 2 P.M. or the week after that on Monday at 10 A.M., would either of those work for you?"

It can be a temptation to adjust your schedule for those who say they cannot see you at any other time. However, when you stretch your schedule to offer times, these very clients may turn out to be unreliable or suddenly request a different time due to a new scheduling problem. Many clients have chaotic, unpredictable lives, and some may unconsciously test limits regardless of your availability. With these possibilities in mind, consider that disrupting your work hours may not be worth it, especially if you are forgoing important down-time you need. Although you may lose some potential clients due to scheduling problems, you gain the opportunity to fill spots with other new clients who can see you during your available times.

My former office mate, Karen, experienced this when a new client asked for a late night appointment well past Karen's normal working hours. She was compelled by this young woman's distress after a recent break-up with her boyfriend, and gave up her one free evening to come back to the office just to see her. Soon into the first session she realized this woman had a long history of instability in many areas of her life; in fact, that very hour she asked to change her appointment time again because she had just decided to reconcile with her boyfriend and wanted to spend nights with him. From that appointment on, Karen guarded her free evenings like a hawk, never scheduling a session during the time she needed for rest and rejuvenation.

Keep in mind that when people are in significant distress and/or highly motivated for therapy, they can often arrange their schedule to fit your available times. This can also be a good indication of their readiness to work in therapy. Even busy professionals and full-time caregivers can use the following strategies successfully to make time for appointments. Those working the traditional 9 A.M. to 5 P.M. hours could use their lunch hour or move lunch to a different time (e.g., an office manager could take lunch at 1 p.m. and use the hour for weekly therapy sessions). Others could arrive to work earlier or stay later, or request leave time (e.g., a school nurse could leave work an hour earlier on therapy days). People in self-employed, management, sales, or other autonomous jobs could shift their activities (e.g., a pharmaceutical sales rep could schedule therapy after lunch appointments). Parents at home full-time could set up reciprocal babysitting with neighbors or friends who also have children at home.

Even with these options, you will encounter some clients who cannot see you within your schedule. In these cases, you can ensure they get the service they need by referring them to fellow clinicians. As I stated earlier, remember to ask clients to share that you have referred them, increasing the chances of reciprocal referrals from your colleagues in the future.

Directions

Once you agree on a time for the initial appointment, you can share your address, directions to your office, and parking options. Giving driving and parking directions to a new client may seem inconsequential, but take a moment to consider your practice location as well as your clientele. If your practice is in an urban area or unfamiliar location, driving to your office the first time could in itself be very stressful due to traffic, and navigating unknown streets. Add to that the distress your clients are already experiencing and it is no simple task to arrive at a first appointment. By taking the time to give specific and detailed directions, you can reduce clients' distress in getting to your office and help them arrive on time at the right place for their first appointments.

You can start with, "I will give you my address and directions to my office. Do you have a pen and paper handy?" Once they do, give them the full address clearly. Clients in great distress often have poor short-term memory and are easily distracted. Spelling the street name and repeating the city ensures that they receive the correct information. Then proceed with, "Where will you be coming from?" Based on clients' answers, you can give driving tips tailored to their starting point. If you can, choose major streets that are easy to find and descriptive landmarks as visual cues along the way. For example, I always include a nearby bridge and marina as references. Cross streets, popular, local businesses, and distinctive building features are additional helpful aides.

A prospective client of mine, Ellen, shared that she suffered from many chronic illnesses and that some days her pain was almost intolerable. Even so, she still drove to all her appointments, so I gave her directions and hoped she would feel well enough the day of her first session. About ten minutes into her session she still hadn't shown up, and when she didn't answer my call, I began to worry. After twenty minutes had passed, I was paged with a message from her; fortunately she was okay and not in too much pain. However, she had gotten lost and was driving in a completely different city looking for my office. Upon calling her back on her cell phone, we soon realized that she had remembered the name Anaheim that I had given her, and assumed that my office was in the city of Anaheim, when I was really referring to a local street named Anaheim. After safely directing her to my office, I resolved to always repeat my city name to clients and to avoid referencing that confusing street name again.

Next, give parking information, reviewing alternative choices in case all spaces are taken. If there are kiosks, gates, fees, or other special features, advise clients in advance what to expect and any special procedures to follow. For clients using public transportation, share nearby transit stops and direct them to their local bus, subway, or other transportation center for specific instructions.

Be sure to get the client's full name, address, and appropriate contact numbers for quick access: "So I can get this down correctly, could you spell your first and last name? Could you also tell me your address and phone numbers that are okay for me to reach you at? Are there certain times that are better or worse to call?"

Paperwork
At this point in the conversation cover any other special instructions, including advising clients to come early to do paperwork. For example, if

you do not have an office manager you might say, "Please arrive twenty minutes early as I will have papers for you to fill out in the waiting room. Because there is no receptionist they will be sitting on the table with my name on them. This will give you time to finish them before our session starts so we can talk about what's going on." Even if clients still arrive late, they will already be informed of the need to finish the paperwork first.

Some clinicians send initial paperwork to clients, instructing them to complete it in advance and bring it to their first session. If you decide to do this, honor confidentiality by making sure their address is private and secure. To help people find your office, you could also include a map of your location. For clients using insurance instruct them to bring their insurance card so you can make a copy.

Issue	Recommendation
Scheduling initial appointments, giving directions, and completing paperwork.	1) To reserve peak-time appointments for clients with limited availability, ask new clients if their schedules are flexible, offering non-peak open times whenever possible (p. 92). 2) To avoid stressful overextensions, if clients ask for times outside your schedule, share your practice hours and offer only current openings; to help clients accommodate to available times, suggest strategies they can use to free up time for appointments (pp. 92–93). 3) To reduce clients' distress in coming to your office and help them arrive on time, offer specific directions with your address, along with parking information (pp. 93–94). 4) To ensure paperwork is done before the initial session begins, direct clients to arrive early to complete this task (pp. 94–95).

Cancellation Policy

The next important issue to cover in the initial conversation is your cancellation policy (see Chapter 8). By having a written policy and explaining it in your phone call, you can fully inform clients that they need to cancel sessions in advance or they will incur a charge for missed visits. This will help reduce last-minute cancellations and no-shows, and allow you enough time to schedule other clients in times that become available. For example, my general explanation is, "There is also a 24-hour cancellation policy. If for some reason you are not able to make the appointment, as long as you let me know more than 24 hours ahead of time, that is fine. However, if you do not, and you don't make it to the appointment,—unfortunately insurance does not pay for missed sessions and—you will be responsible for the entire amount of _____ dollars, not just the co-pay for the missed visit. You seem like a very responsible person and I don't expect this to come up, but I wanted to let you know the policy right away just in case. Do you anticipate any problems with this?" You will probably find that most people are familiar with cancellation policies and quickly agree to call ahead if something comes up.

When starting in practice, although I included my cancellation policy in the consent form I gave to clients to fill out when they arrived at my office, I did not review it during the phone call before the first appointment. I found that a number of first-time clients did not make it to their initial appointment. Because they had not yet read about the policy in the consent form, they usually called to cancel at the last minute, leaving no time to offer the spot to someone else. After I started explaining the cancellation policy over the phone, I noticed a significant drop in the number of no-shows and last-minute cancellations. Consider, too, that clients are often nervous and ambivalent about seeking help. A cancellation policy can provide the extra boost they need to follow through in making it to their appointments, especially if they get cold feet at the last minute.

Reminders

Before finishing the call, again remind clients who need insurance authorization, "As we discussed before, please call your insurance company back right away to tell them our first appointment time and complete the authorization. Then, please call me back with the authorization number, the number of visits covered, and your co-pay. This will make sure your visits are covered by your insurance."

After this reminder, write a note to yourself to call their insurance company a day or two before the first visit to see whether the authorization has been completed. If precertification has not been done, you can either do it yourself or give clients another reminder call to do this. Although you can usually initiate the first authorization with insurance directly, I have found that when clients do it themselves certifications are often more generous than when I have asked. Plus, by being actively involved in securing their own treatment, a client's motivation and investment in ongoing therapy will likely increase.

To finish the call, review the appointment and payment one more time, "So I'll look forward to meeting you Thursday August 12th at 3 P.M., and again your fee is _____ dollars. Do you have any last questions?" If so, you can respond right away with answers that are compatible with your practice parameters, comfort level, and working style. If clients don't have any, you can also address common questions yourself, educating them about your practice well in advance of their first session.

POSSIBLE LAST-MINUTE CLIENT REQUESTS TO ADDRESS

- Asking to bring a baby or small child to individual sessions.
- Showing up with spouses, other family members, roommates, etc., and asking if they can attend clients' individual sessions.
- Asking to bring an older child who has behavioral and/or emotional problems that would be disruptive to sessions to sit in the waiting room.
- Coming to appointments when ill and contagious and requesting to stay.
- Appearing for appointments after drinking or abusing drugs.
- Asking if it's okay to stay parked in a handicapped or other assigned parking space.

Although there are other questions and issues that might arise, one question I am sometimes asked is if clients can bring their baby or small child to their individual session. A number of my clients are primary caregivers with no other childcare resources in place. Early in my practice I granted this request and quickly found it to be detrimental to therapy. I remember one mother describing with confidence her six-month-old Zachary's calm temperament. Upon arriving to the session Zachary cried intermittently to the very end and his mother kept shaking her head, baffled by this new behavior, all of which restricted our therapeutic progress.

Since then I have answered clients by saying, "Unfortunately I don't have childcare facilities in my office and your child will not be able to come to the session. Although it may not seem like it, even small babies can be affected by what goes on in the session, and to protect them from negative effects they should not be present. Also, attending to your child can distract both of us and take away from our work together. This time is yours and you deserve to have it completely to yourself with no interruptions. For these reasons you'll need to make arrangements for childcare."

Although most parents ask first before bringing children, I've also had clients who just show up to their first appointment with children in tow. One mother brought her two-year-old daughter, Courtney, who was fascinated by the water fountain, and the entire session was consumed with making sure Courtney was safe and did not break anything. These situations were stressful and disruptive for everyone, taking time and energy to discuss the problem and decide whether to proceed or reschedule the session. Now if I become aware that a client is a stay-at-home parent or primary caregiver, I address this issue on the phone before the first appointment to avoid a stressful surprise.

In your practice these requests may not be frequent or they may not apply to your style of work (e.g., you may be comfortable providing therapy for individuals who bring children or you may exclusively do family or child therapy where children are always present). By identifying potentially stressful requests common to your practice, you can proactively address them, preventing problems before they have a chance to surface.

Issue	Recommendation
Reviewing your cancellation policy and reminders before the first session.	1) To reduce last-minute cancellations and no-shows, establish a cancellation policy and explain it to clients over the phone before the first session (pp. 95–96). 2) To ensure that services are covered by insurance, remind clients to complete authorizations and call back with the details; check before the first visit to make sure this gets done (pp. 96–97). 3) To wrap up calls, review appointment details and ask for any final questions; to prevent common problems from surfacing during initial appointments, address them over the phone, educating clients regarding your practice limits before the first session (pp. 97–98).

CHAPTER FIVE

Verifying Insurance Benefits Efficiently

After setting initial appointments and finishing phone calls with insured clients, the next important step is to contact their insurance companies as soon as possible to verify benefits. If dealing with insurance sounds unpleasant to you, I definitely share your sentiment; I would rate it as one of my least favorite tasks in private practice. Insurance systems are replete with many hoops to jump through and ever-changing rules to follow before you are finally paid for services. They have separate departments for authorizations, benefits, customer service, billing, etc.; this compartmentalized structure is ripe for miscommunication, lost information (especially authorizations and claims), and denied payments. And anytime companies upgrade computer systems or have high staff turnover, mistakes are even more likely. It would be easier if every insurance provider operated similarly, but they do not; each dictates its own requirements, especially for managed care plans.

Confirm Coverage in Advance

Given these formidable challenges, your best approach when working with insurance companies is to follow a proactive plan to protect your clients and your practice. This chapter offers such a plan, guiding you through the specific steps necessary to obtain valid authorizations and benefits. By confirming coverage details, you can fully inform clients of their exact payment in advance, giving them the time they may need to solve any problems in securing the funds. You will also be able to alert them if their insurance does not cover your services, giving you time to discuss an alternate self-pay option or to make referrals to other affordable services. Whatever roadblocks may surface, following the plan outlined will afford you and your clients the time to deal with them before the first session, avoiding the stress and financial drain of starting therapy and then finding out the client can't continue because of payment or benefit problems.

Although you will be verifying benefits, keep in mind that it is your clients' responsibility to know their benefits and pay any fees that insurance does not cover. Clients may not remember that you covered this in the inquiry call; during the second phone call, when sharing benefit and payment information, remind them again so they will be fully informed that these items are ultimately their responsibility.

My colleague, Sara, learned the value of confirming insurance coverage when starting to see clients in her solo practice. She had completed the process of becoming a contracted provider with five insurance companies and was certain that she could see clients covered through these plans. Soon after, a prospective client named Kim called to request services for panic attacks and stressful conflicts with her boyfriend. These presenting issues were compatible with her services, so Sara proceeded to ask questions about insurance coverage. Kim planned to use her insurance benefits to pay for sessions and Sara was pleased to hear the client's carrier was Blue Cross, one of the five companies with whom she had just contracted to provide services. Kim hadn't called for a referral and did not know what her payment responsibilities were, but Sara was certain that Blue Cross did not require precertification for these services and paid a large percentage of billed fees.

Sara was so eager to provide services that she did not ask for identifying information on Kim's insurance card or call to verify benefits. She guessed that Kim's co-pay would be about twenty dollars, which Kim was pleased to hear. She scheduled Kim for the first available appointment the next day and when Kim arrived, Sara followed her routine of copying Kim's insurance card to place in her file. As she turned the Blue Cross card over to copy the other side, she glanced at the information and could not believe what she saw in small text: "For mental health benefits call PacifiCare 1-800-000-0000." To make matters worse, PacifiCare was not one of the five companies with whom she had contracted. Sara was now facing the aversive task of calling to learn that mental health coverage was handled through PacifiCare, which paid only for precertified treatment given by in-network providers. Meanwhile Kim was waiting for her in the next room with sweaty palms, a racing heart, and completely absorbed by her last argument with her boyfriend.

Sara explained the situation to Kim, called PacifiCare to confirm the unwelcome news that she would not be paid for services, and discussed options for continued care. Kim could not afford services on her own, even at a discount, and chose to see another therapist contracted through PacifiCare. Sara helped her call PacifiCare for a referral, and stayed with Kim as she called the new therapist to set up the first appointment. These efforts took the entire session, and at the end Kim was feeling better and looking forward to seeing her new therapist the next day. Sara was glad that Kim would be able to continue with affordable care, but was appalled at how much time, income, and energy she lost setting things up for a new client and not being able to continue offering treatment. She resolved to never again skip the insurance benefit check before first sessions, no matter how straightforward the coverage initially appeared.

Tailor Steps to Your Practice

When reading the following steps, it may seem like you have a lot to do, but in practice you can complete benefit verification very quickly. You can also modify steps to suit your individual practice needs, skipping any questions that don't apply. And once you become familiar with standard benefits and authorization rules of insurance providers, you can tailor questions to each one, further shortening the benefit check. As you get used to your individualized protocol, the process can take as little as a minute or two, especially when you get through to an agent right away. For example, in my practice, many of my clients are covered through just a few different insurance companies whose benefits I now know pretty well. When calling these carriers, in just a few questions I gain all the benefit and authorization information I need.

Trend to Reduce Precertification

A welcome development that may further streamline your task is a growing trend among managed care companies toward fewer precertification requirements. Some companies are now granting more visits per request compared to previous years; many have simplified from multi- to one-page outpatient treatment request forms (OTRs). I remember years ago receiving bulky packets filled with lengthy OTRs that had pages of open-ended essay questions to complete for future certification requests. Now I usually get a one-page OTR with boxes to check. And while I was writing this chapter, one company, Cigna, set a precedent by completely eliminating preauthorization for sessions. If this trend continues, you may be able to forego many or all of the precertification issues. Keep alert to any changes in your insurance companies' policies, often when one changes, others will follow.

Calling Tips

Several phone practices will help you to efficiently verify clients' benefits. They include using a speakerphone, preserving private numbers, making direct contact, identifying yourself, and recording your contact.

Use a Speakerphone

When calling to verify insurance benefits, consider using a speakerphone (or a headset, or earpiece) so that if you are placed on hold, you can complete other tasks during this otherwise wasted time. Since you will be shifting your attention back and forth between these activities and your calls, select chores that do not require much concentration (e.g., copying and filing) as opposed to more challenging mental tasks, such as writing reports. When I am on hold, I usually go through junk mail, check my schedule, organize client charts for the next day, review other calls to make, and see whether any authorization requests are due.

Preserve Your Privacy

After reaching insurance agents, one of the first things they may do is ask for the phone number you are calling from for their records. Be sure to always give your public work number even if you are calling from home or somewhere else. This will reduce the chances of your private number being circulated and possibly ending up in unintended hands (e.g., clients). Most companies 800 numbers automatically identify where you are calling from; by always stating your work number, your chances are greater that this public number will be recorded by the agent, overriding any initially detected private number and preserving your confidentiality. Remember to do this even if you have complete caller ID blocking, because, as I stated earlier, this privacy feature is automatically overridden every time you make a toll-free call.

Make Direct Contact

Calls to insurance companies can lead to recorded messages and delays before you reach an agent to whom you can pose your questions. It may be tempting to choose the automated option to receive benefit information, as this may seem to be the easiest and fastest way to learn about covered services. Or newer, online options may appeal; checking benefits through insurance companies' websites. However, you run the risk of receiving incorrect information and you have no way to immediately ask questions or clarify details. By talking directly with an insurance agent you can ask specific questions about mental health coverage and gain complete, current, and accurate benefit information.

I learned the value of making direct contact with agents soon after starting in practice. Thinking I would save time, I called an insurance carrier's automated system to hear benefits for a prospective client, a depressed mother overwhelmed with the responsibilities of caring for her three children under the age of five. The recording said she was eligible for services, quoted a low co-payment, and made no mention of a deductible or pre-certification required for mental health services. Fortunately, I then called to confirm this information directly with an agent, as these benefits sounded too good to be true. Sure enough, the mental health coverage was handled by a completely different company requiring preauthorization for services to be paid. The carrier also had different in- and out-of-network benefits; if the client chose a non-contracted therapist she would have to pay a high deductible and tiered co-payments.

Luckily, I was contracted with this second mental health company and the client was able to receive services from me at a low co-payment rate with no deductible. However, if I had not directly verified benefits with an agent and I was not an in-network provider, my overwhelmed client would have learned of unexpected payments due well after starting therapy, likely adding to her depression and impeding therapy progress. Moreover, I would have been faced with the difficult task of telling her this unwelcome news and attempting to collect additional payments due.

Identify Yourself

Typically the insurance company's phone number you receive from clients is a general customer service number, and when calling it you will probably hear a recorded menu of choices. Choose the option for providers and then eligibility/benefits to speak directly with a customer service agent. If you get stuck in a prerecorded maze, try pressing 0; this will often route you to a live person. After reaching someone, identify yourself right away, "This is Dr. Roberts, licensed psychologist, and I am calling to receive outpatient mental health benefits for a new patient." Whomever you reach will then know what you need and be able to direct you to the appropriate benefit agent. By specifically stating your professional connection to the client, you are more likely to receive helpful answers and extra consideration than if you do not give this kind of information. Even if you don't generally refer to clients as patients, it helps to do so when talking with insurance agents; I have found them to be especially responsive to medical model terms.

Record Your Contact

You may be directed to another number right away, as different companies often have exclusive contracts to handle mental health benefits. If so, write down the new number for future reference. As a general rule when calling insurance providers, always record every contact by writing down the date you called, the insurance company name and phone number, the agent's full name (or first name and first initial of their last name), his/her phone number and extension, and any specific information you can obtain. This creates a trail of accountability if you are ever quoted something incorrectly and need to show evidence of the error. This written record can be critical if you are denied payment for services; you will be able to quickly trace back to the source of the problem. By sharing details of the error including the agent's name, date of contact, and incorrect information, you are much more likely to receive assistance in correcting any denied claim than if you rely on your general request for payment alone. Your written record in many cases could mean the difference between being paid or not for your services.

Issue	Recommendation
Calling insurance carriers to verify clients' benefits.	1) To efficiently use time when you are on hold during benefit verification calls, use a speakerphone (headset, earpiece) and choose simple tasks to do (p. 102). 2) To preserve the privacy of your confidential number when calling toll-free insurance numbers, always state your public work number to agents (pp. 102–103). 3) To avoid receiving incorrect benefit information, speak directly with insurance agents to verify coverage details (p. 103). 4) To reach insurance agents for benefit checks, choose the provider and benefits/eligibility options; to enhance quality service, always state your professional identity and relationship to the client (p. 104). 5) To provide a written record of accountability to which you can refer to correct any payment problems, always record every contact with insurance agents (p. 104).

General Tips

Several practices will facilitate accurate and comprehensive insurance benefit quotes. They include sharing identifying information, confirming mental health coverage, checking for parity benefits and comparing quotes to your expectations.

Share Identifying Information

You will next be asked for the client's identifying information, usually starting with the insured's name, the subscriber ID number from the insurance card, the client's name, and birth date. You may also be asked for the insured's employer name, and group number. This should be the same information you have already obtained from your client during the initial phone call.

Confirm Mental Health Coverage

When verifying coverage, make sure you receive specific mental health benefit information. Agents can easily forget your initial request for mental health benefits and instead quote the more commonly requested medical coverage out of habit. These mistakes can create many problems later since medical benefits are often more generous than mental health benefits. For example, mental health benefits are more likely to require preauthorization of services, the use of in-network providers, and substantial co-payments compared to medical benefits. When your agent reviews coverage, if it sounds too good to be true, you could be hearing medical and not mental health benefits.

To prevent this from happening ask the insurance agent, "Are you certain these are mental health and not general medical benefits?" If yes, "Are you certain these are mental health benefits for non-MD providers? I am an L.P.C. [licensed professional counselor]" or "I am a Ph.D., licensed psychologist" or "I am an L.C.S.W., licensed social worker—will these benefits still apply?" Sometimes mental health coverage is further restricted based on licensure, so this specific question allows you to confirm whether services you provide and bill through your license will be paid.

My colleague, Susan, experienced this firsthand when an insurance company denied her services for payment. She had called in advance to verify benefits, talked directly with an agent, and asked all the right questions. However, the one question she didn't ask was whether services billed through her marriage and family therapist (MFT) license would be paid. The agent made no mention of this restriction, instead quoting details such as deductible, co-payment, and yearly benefit limits. Only after receiving insurance denials for weeks of therapy services did Susan learn of this problem. This insurance carrier was based in another state that did not have MFT licensure, and thus did not recognize her license as eligible for reimbursement. Her billed services would only have been paid if she were licensed as a social worker, psychologist, or psychiatrist. Unfortunately, by the time she found this out her clients had stopped therapy and did not respond to her attempts to collect payment. After that distressing experience, Susan resolved to always confirm that her license is eligible for payment when calling new insurance carriers she has not worked with before. She has successfully avoided this problem ever since.

Check for Parity Benefits

In recent years many states have passed parity laws granting certain severe mental illnesses the same insurance coverage as other medical conditions.

For example, California enacted parity legislation in 2000 whereby patients with severe illnesses such as bipolar, panic, and major depressive disorder receive benefits matching those covering other medical illnesses. If your state has a parity law, find out what diagnoses are covered and then routinely ask for non-parity (basic) and parity (deluxe) quotes when verifying each patient's insurance: "Does this patient's insurance include parity benefits? Could you please give me benefit quotes for both parity and non-parity diagnoses?" Since you probably won't know before meeting clients who has parity diagnoses and who does not, having both benefit quotes will allow you to later match the appropriate benefits after you have established your clients' diagnoses in person. Some agents may ask you for the patient's diagnosis; if so you can say you don't know because you haven't met the patient yet.

Compare Quotes To Your Expectations

If you accept managed care insurance, you may quickly become familiar with their standard benefits and authorization procedures, especially of the companies you work with the most. If the past trend of mergers and takeovers continue, you will also have fewer companies to keep straight.

Issue	Recommendation
Facilitating accurate and comprehensive benefit quotes.	1) To allow insurance agents quick access to clients' benefits, tell them the identifying information clients gave you from their insurance cards (p. 105). 2) To ensure that you receive correct benefit information, ask agents to confirm that coverage is specifically for mental health, and that services billed through your license will be paid (p. 106). 3) To receive comprehensive benefit quotes, find out whether your state has enacted a parity law; if so, find out what diagnoses are covered and routinely ask for parity and non-parity benefit quotes, applying the correct benefit after diagnosing your client (pp. 106–107). 4) To ensure correct benefit quotes for insurance plans you work with often, compare information you receive with past quotes, addressing and correcting any discrepancies (pp. 107–108).

Whenever I call an insurance provider I work with often, I compare the benefit quote to my expectations based on past experience. If there is a discrepancy, I pursue it further to make sure there are no errors. This can work to your advantage even when you find no mistakes. For example, once during a routine benefit check for a new client, the agent shared that an initial certification had been done for five sessions, not the ten that I was used to receiving. When I pointed this out, she said they had just reduced the standard number authorized to all providers from ten to five, but since I asked she would certify ten. As this experience shows, it never hurts to point out inconsistencies you encounter, especially to advocate for your clients; you may just free yourself from some paperwork as well.

Areas to Cover During Benefit Checks

By covering several crucial areas during insurance benefit checks, you can ensure comprehensive and accurate benefit/payment quotes. The following protocol guides you in addressing these areas, providing you with the specific questions to ask agents during insurance benefit checks.

1) Network Status   5) Co-Payment
2) Benefit Maximums   6) Deductible
3) Services Covered   7) Billing
4) Precertification

Often when agents quote benefits, they start with a disclaimer that the benefit summary does not guarantee payment; the patient must be eligible at the time services are rendered, and other requirements specific to the insurance must be met (e.g., provider is contracted with the insurance carrier, certification has been done). They usually tell you the patient's effective date (when he/she first became eligible for services with that insurance), the total number of visits allowed per year, and the patient's payment responsibility. Whatever the initial quote, much crucial data will probably be left out. To confirm benefits, make sure agents cover the following areas before finishing your call.

Network Status

"Is this an Indemnity, PPO, EPO, POS, or HMO plan?" The type of plan your client is covered by will give you a quick idea of the extent of benefits.

Indemnity plans are typically the most generous and least restrictive and HMO plans are the least generous and most restrictive. Indemnity plans generally allow subscribers to choose their own providers, do not require precertification, and offer high benefit limits (e.g., fifty or more sessions per year). Preferred provider (PPO), exclusive provider (EPO), and point-of-service (POS) plans either require or encourage subscribers to receive in-network care, paying a higher portion of fees if subscribers see contracted as opposed to non-contracted providers. Some of these plans require precertification and benefit limits are typically less compared to indemnity plans (e.g., thirty to forty sessions per year). Health maintenance organization (HMO) plans restrict service to in-network providers only, usually require precertification, and typically offer the lowest benefit limits (e.g., ten to twenty sessions per year).

"Does this plan require in-network providers?" PPO, EPO, POS, and HMO plans often restrict payment to contracted providers. If yes, ask, *"Am I listed as an in-network provider?"* The agent can usually search the provider database by asking for your name, address, tax ID number, and any other provider ID specific to the company. For insurance plans that you work with often and are certain you are contracted with as a provider, you may decide to skip this question. However, if you are newly contracted or change your practice, verify that the insurance provider's listing is updated correctly and that you are currently an active in-network provider. Do this whenever you move, add a second location, change phone numbers, or transition from a group to an individual practice. Anytime you change information, errors could cause your name and practice data to be inadvertently erased or dropped from the network. If you check your provider status before seeing a new client and there is a problem, you can deal with it right away, avoiding the costly experience of having your claims denied because you are not an in-network provider.

My colleague, Jennifer, assumed that since she was already contracted with a managed care company, her services would automatically be covered for any new client with this insurance. She was working in a group practice that routinely handled benefits and billing, and had just decided to sublet office space one day a week in another city with the goal to develop an individual practice there.

A psychiatrist colleague referred a woman with generalized anxiety and a severe phobia of ants to Jennifer. It was summer—a heavy season for ant problems—and this woman was extremely anxious and in great need of services. Jennifer was pleased when this client told her she had coverage through an insurance carrier that Jennifer had contracted with, and proceeded to schedule a first session at her new office location.

She then called the insurance provider to check this client's benefits and was shocked when she was told that although she was contracted with this company, the contract was through her group practice only, and she was not able to bill for services as an individual provider. She learned that in order to bill for services individually, she would need to contract again as an individual provider, a process that could take months. If Jennifer had seen this client at her new office location and billed through her individual practice identifiers before clarifying the situation, all services would have been denied for payment.

If you are not a contracted provider, ask, *"Does this patient have out-of-network benefits?"* If so, the client can see you even if you are not on the network panel. *"What are the benefits?"* Usually clients will need to pay more in the form of a higher deductible and co-pays, there may be fewer visits allowed, and other restrictions may apply. Whatever the limitations, these benefits are still important to know and relay to clients; they may still choose to see you, especially if someone they trust has personally referred them.

Yearly and Lifetime Maximums

"How many visits are allowed each year?" You will be better able to plan treatment when you know session limits in advance. *"What is the maximum dollar amount covered each year?"* If there are unlimited visits, there are usually monetary caps. *"What benefits have already been used this year?"* Some new clients will have already seen other therapists, and this answer will tell you just how much of their benefit is left to cover your services. If clients see a psychiatrist regularly as well, these visits also typically count toward yearly mental health benefits.

One of my new clients with severe depression and anxiety had been to her psychiatrist five times that year for medication checks before calling in April for her first appointment with me. Her benefit covered thirty mental health sessions every calendar year, including psychiatrist visits. By telling her of these limits, we could plan treatment, accounting for psychiatrist visits, and review options in the event that her benefits were exhausted before December.

We agreed to start with weekly sessions, and depending on progress, spread visits out to ensure continued care, which we did around September. However, in November her symptoms increased as the holidays approached and she had more contact with her dysfunctional family. She requested weekly sessions and because she was nearing her thirty-visit limit, she was fully prepared to pay cash for the few weeks of sessions before her benefits renewed in January. Having ascertained her insurance limitations before beginning treatment, we avoided the unpleasant surprise of her having to suddenly pay for uncovered visits.

"What is the lifetime maximum number of sessions?" On occasion you may find a very restrictive plan (e.g., a lifetime limit of fifty sessions). *"What is the lifetime maximum amount covered?"* This can be important if the cap is unusually low and you do long-term therapy, as amounts can add up fast. In general you will find that carriers offer adequate lifetime benefits.

Services Covered

"Are any diagnoses excluded from payment?" Insurance carriers usually exclude coverage for personality disorders and V code conditions (problems not severe enough to fit the criteria for diagnoses). Some companies do not pay for select diagnoses within categories, such as attention-deficit, disruptive behavior, and learning disorders.

"Is (marital therapy) a covered benefit?" If you plan to provide services that could fall outside standard coverage (e.g., couples and family therapy, psychological testing, drug and alcohol treatment, hypnosis), specifically ask if those services are covered. If the service is covered, make sure all benefit questions are addressed. You may be asked to provide a corresponding CPT (Current Procedural Terminology) code, which is a standard billing identifier, so it's good to know them for each service you provide. If you are contracted with any insurance panels, these codes will usually be listed on your fee schedules and/or in your provider manuals. Unlike medical services, mental health services have just a few codes so you won't have too many to remember. For instance, my typical bills include just one or two codes. You can also obtain a complete CPT coding manual, published and updated regularly by the American Medical Association (available at www.psych.org).

My former office mate, Denise, specializes in marital therapy and on occasion she learns that prospective clients' insurance plans do not cover this service. Anytime she provides couples counseling, she thoroughly checks the spouse's insurance benefits; often both people have different insurance policies. She usually finds that one plan does cover marital therapy and can bill services through that company, allowing clients to use their benefits in utilizing her services.

"This patient is also insured by another policy, is this insurance primary and should it be billed first?" If your client is covered by two insurance policies and you bill both, you will need to determine which one is your client's primary carrier and bill that one first. Clients usually know which policy is primary, but to be sure you should ask the agent. For example, sometimes Denise learns that her client does not have coverage for marital therapy on his/her primary policy. Instead, the marital therapy is covered by the client's secondary policy. Denise must first bill the primary carrier, receive a payment denial statement, and then bill the secondary carrier with the attached denial from the first insurance company.

important

Precertification

"Do visits require precertification?" Even companies you are certain don't require this can quickly change their rules. If authorization is required and you do not obtain it, you can be denied payment with little recourse to recoup your lost income.

"Has precertification already been done for the patient to see me?" If yes, *"What is the approval number?"* Most companies require these approval numbers to be put on claims when billing for services.

"How many sessions have been approved?" Some companies are more generous (e.g., ten to twenty) and others grant just a few at a time (e.g., three to five). *"What is the timeframe to use them?"* This can range from very short (e.g., one to three months) to very long (e.g., one year or open-ended). *"What are the allowed CPT codes for these services?"* Make sure they match the services you are planning to provide. Some companies allow a CPT code of 90801 (initial evaluation) for the first session, which are usually paid at a higher rate by insurance carriers, while others do not.

"Will a certification letter be sent to me?" Large insurance companies sometimes lose this information or fail to send it to the correct billing departments, resulting in—you guessed it—payment denials. When you have a written or electronic record of the authorization from the insurance company, you can more easily prove that services were approved and should be paid. If any company does not offer certification acknowledgments, record the name of the agent you talked with, the time and day of your contact, and all certification details. If there is a discrepancy and/or denial of payment, you can reference this evidence of approval and more easily facilitate reimbursement.

After an insurance company denied many hours of service I had billed, I called the billing agent who explained that there was no record of an authorization for these services. Fortunately I found a copy of the certification letter in the client's file, clearly showing that approval had been performed. I informed the agent, who directed me to re-bill for the services with a copy of the authorization attached. Although it took another month between re-billing to payment, I was reimbursed for every service because I had proof that the authorization had been completed.

If certification is required and has not been done, ask *"What is the process to precertify?"* Be sure to get a phone number to call and find out whether you or the client should request certification. Some plans will only allow the client to initiate treatment; if you learn of this requirement at the last minute, you can still direct clients to call during the first session to ensure insurance payments for the visit. Clients will be grateful that you caught this and will be happy to request certification to avoid paying an extra fee, even if it takes up some session time.

If for some reason you start seeing a client and then find out precertification was required, you or your clients can call and request a retroactive authorization to cover prior sessions. If you call first and are denied, ask your client to make the same request. Insurance companies may be more likely to accommodate a concerned policyholder as opposed to a licensed provider. If this does not work, you can usually file a written appeal requesting payment for denied sessions. Although you can often retroactively fix certification problems, you will save yourself much grief and time by completing authorizations before seeing clients.

"What is the process to request future certifications?" Companies have varying procedures when requesting additional sessions. Some send a treatment request form with the initial authorization letter, directing you to complete and send it before the final approved session. Others do phone reviews following a protocol outlined in their provider manual. Many insurance carriers now allow you to request sessions through their websites. Some require the client to also complete a questionnaire and send it before future sessions are granted.

By learning procedures specific to each company, you can plan your treatment requests, noting when it's time to ask for more sessions, what method you need to use, and whether you need to remind the client to do anything. By following this process, you can ensure uninterrupted treatment and payment for all sessions.

My former office neighbor, Joan, encountered a different requirement when working with Jane, a full-time college student. Jane was a young adult woman suffering from depression, and was covered through her parents' managed care insurance policy. Joan was a preferred provider with this company and was very familiar with the certification process. However, she wasn't aware until receiving her first payment denial that Jane was required to show proof of full-time student status every semester in order to be eligible for benefits. After learning of this requirement, she directed Jane to give her a copy of the completed registration for every semester, including summer. Sometimes this was no easy task, as Jane would forget to bring her class schedule when her depressive symptoms were severe. Joan started reminding Jane of this task weeks before a new semester would start. This was well worth the effort, as once Joan received each registration, she routinely sent a copy with every bill, preventing future payment denials.

Co-Payment

"What is the patient's co-payment per session?" You may get a fixed number, such as fifteen or twenty dollars, or a quote of a percentage whereby part is paid by insurance and the remaining percent the client pays. If you are contracted with any insurance companies, these percentages are based on your contracted rates (allowed amounts), which are usually lower than your normal rates. To prevent charging clients too much, use your contracted rates to calculate exactly what clients owe. For example, if your session rate is $100, you are contracted with an insurance company to accept an allowed amount of eighty dollars, and insurance pays 80 percent, the client's co-pay is 20 percent of eighty dollars or sixteen dollars per session. If you don't know what your contracted rate is for the insurance plan in question, you can look it up in your contract files or call the company's provider relations department.

"Does the co-payment increase as more visits are used?" Insurance plans sometimes have tiered client payment rates: for example, nothing for the first five visits, ten dollars for visits six through ten, and twenty-five dollars for visits eleven through fifty. If so, ask, *"Does this co-payment schedule start over at the beginning of the year or any time during the year?"* Most plans reset every calendar year (January 1); a few renew at the first of a different month. Some plans do not start over, extending the same co-payment schedule until the end of a treatment episode.

Deductible

"Is there a deductible?" A deductible is the amount a client must first pay out of pocket each year before insurance starts paying for services. Agents often overlook this crucial detail when quoting benefits. If there is a deductible there's a good chance clients have not yet met the limit. If you don't find out, you will receive unpaid insurance claims whenever your billed amounts are applied toward deductibles. You will also be the bearer of unhappy news when you bill clients for these unexpected fees. Most indemnity, EPO, and PPO plans do have a deductible and many of them are quite high. Although typically managed care plans do not charge a deductible if clients see a contracted provider, some do, so ask to be sure.

"Does this deductible apply to both medical and mental health services?" Once in a while insurance companies will have a separate deductible for medical and mental health services. If so, proceed with questions specific to the mental health deductible.

"How much is the deductible?" and *"How much has already been paid?"* Different plans have different amounts; by obtaining the exact deductible and knowing how much remains, you can calculate how much clients need to pay you for each visit until their deductible is met.

"Is this a calendar year deductible or does it start over at a different time in the year?" Although most deductibles renew the first day of January, some reset on a different month (similar to tiered co-pays). Relaying this to clients will help them budget for the deductible expense before it starts over each year. Some prospective clients with a large unpaid deductible who call close to renewal may choose to delay services to avoid paying the deductible expense twice. Other clients in immediate crisis may choose to proceed regardless of the cost. Whatever their unique situation, clients will appreciate this information and be better able to plan payments for services, avoiding unexpected financial stress.

Stacy, a potential client, called me in late October to request treatment for depression and low self-esteem. She had been in therapy two years ago and wanted to start services again as she was just beginning to notice the first signs that her depression was returning. At the same time, she was financially strapped; she had just finished an internship in occupational therapy and was working hard to save enough to move to another city to live with her fiancée the following summer.

After conducting the benefit check, I informed Stacy of her $600 deductible, that only $100 had been met so far that year, and that the deductible would start over again in January. She decided that since it was only two months until she could start paying off her deductible for the following year, she was not in crisis and could utilize tools she had gained in prior therapy. She waited until January to schedule her first appointment. She agreed that if her depression worsened, she would call before January to start therapy. With this strategy Stacy was able to save money to help with her future move, and avoided a financial stress that could have increased her depression.

"Are there any claims that have been recently submitted that will reduce the remaining deductible once they are processed?" Often clients have received other medical/mental health care and the claims are not yet fully processed. Once this is done, it may help lower the remaining deductible. Agents can usually estimate the amount of these pending charges that will apply. The more accurate you can be in estimating what clients owe on their deductibles, the more certain you can be of collecting the exact fee at the time of each session, preventing overcharges and the extra work of preparing refunds.

Billing

"What is the billing address to submit mental health claims?" Having the correct address is vital to facilitating claims payments, and it may be entirely different from the one on the client's insurance card. This often occurs when mental health benefits are handled through a different company from the client's medical policy. For example, if the client's medical plan is Blue Shield, United Behavioral Health (UBH) administers the mental health benefits. Although there is a Blue Shield claims address on the insurance card, the correct billing address will be through UBH.

My colleague, Sara, discovered this issue when calling for a benefit check for one of her new clients, Kinisha, a young woman with panic attacks and relationship problems. Kinisha's insurance card said Blue Shield, but when Sara called, the agent advised her that the mental health benefits were handled through Managed Health Network. With this one phone call before Kinisha's first session, Sara was able to preauthorize services, learn accurate benefit information, and obtain the correct billing address to which to send claims. She then told Kinisha her exact payments due for each session, and was able to move on to give full attention to providing the services that Kinisha needed right away.

If you are submitting out-of-network claims ask, *"Is there a different address to which to send out-of-network claims?"* Companies often have separate billing addresses for in-network and out-of-network claims. Anytime you bill the wrong address there will be an extra month or longer delay in your payment while the claim is rerouted, or it could be denied and sent back to you, requiring a repeat billing to the correct claims address.

"What is the phone number for billing and claims questions?" This will be helpful if you run into any payment problems later. *"Is there a special claim form that must be used or can I use the standard HCFA–1500 (Health Care Financing Administration) claim form (UB-92 for in-patient services)?"* On

Issue	Recommendation
Calling clients' insurance carriers to check benefits before their first session.	1) To ensure comprehensive and accurate benefit/payment quotes during benefit checks, follow the protocol on pages 108–117. 2) To assess network rules, ask whether the insurance plan requires in-network providers, and if so, whether you are contracted with that company; if you are not, ask for out-of-network benefits and offer them to clients (pp. 108–110). 3) To aid in treatment planning, find out benefit maximums and any diagnoses that are excluded from payment; ask whether your specific services will be covered and, when applicable, which carrier is primary (pp. 110–112). 4) To ensure insurance payments, find out if precertification is required and whether it has already been done; ask for a confirmation letter and for the specific process to request future certifications (pp. 112–114). 5) To collect correct co-payments from clients, find out their exact amounts due; check for tiered increases and if schedules reset any time during the year (p. 114). 6) To ensure payment for deductibles if required, find out how much remains to be paid, when the deductible(s) starts over again, and if there are any submitted claims that will reduce the deductible(s) once they are processed (pp. 115–116). 7) To facilitate timely claims payments, obtain the billing address to which to send mental health claims; request contact numbers for billing questions, and find out if any special claim form is required (pp. 116–118).

occasion you may find a managed care plan that requires a different claim form from the widely accepted HCFA-1500 form, more recently named the CMS-1500 (Centers for Medicare and Medicaid Services). If you bill on the wrong form, payment will be denied and you'll have to resubmit the claims on the correct form.

Confirm Benefits Every New Year

To ensure continuous and accurate benefits, ask ongoing clients at the first of the year if they have the same insurance plan. If they have received new insurance cards, make a copy for your records and call the carrier again to verify benefits. Even if insurance plans remain the same, specific benefits can change. For example, yearly limits may decrease, deductibles and co-payments may increase, authorization procedures and claims addresses may change, etc. By conducting benefit checks right away after January 1, you can fully inform your clients of these changes, helping them to plan their finances and ensuring appropriate and timely compensation for your services.

A checklist of the specific questions we've covered is included in Appendix C. You may wish to keep a copy available for reference when calling insurance companies for benefit checks.

Confirming Benefits with Clients

If you receive unexpected or new information during the benefit check, call clients as soon as possible to fully inform them in advance of their first session. Although some people may cancel a first appointment if they feel the payment is too high, it is easier on everyone if they do this before investing time and effort in services they will not be able to afford.

When sharing benefit information over the phone, start on a positive note to validate clients' decisions to seek services: "I have some good news, your insurance plan does have mental health benefits and you are able to use them to see me for services." If you think it is too overwhelming or complicated for clients to review all the details over the phone, you can save most of the information to share in person. Just be sure they know the exact payment to bring to the initial session. If you learn of unanticipated expensive deductibles or co-payment schedules, share this too. For any remaining details, be sure to review them in your first meeting to prevent future payment miscommunications or problems. The table below offers specific suggestions on how to optimally communicate benefit information to your clients.

SUGGESTIONS FOR CONFIRMING BENEFITS AND PAYMENT RESPONSIBILITIES

- To fully inform clients and help them assess whether they can afford services, call them right after completing the benefit check with any unexpected payments required.
- To avoid overwhelming clients with complicated benefit information, save most details to share in person; confirm over the phone their exact payment for the first session and any high deductibles or co-payment schedules.
- To prevent disappointing clients if their payments are higher than expected, assume non-parity (basic) benefits until you can establish diagnoses in person.
- To help clients budget for expensive deductibles, share how much they must pay each visit until the total is met; to reduce distress about bills, reassure clients with combined deductibles that insurance will record their payments, and after fulfilling their deductible they will not have to pay it again when receiving any medical or mental health services for the rest of the year.
- To ensure payment for services, collect client portions due at the time of service and bill insurance for the remaining amount.
- To help clients budget for future services, share co-payment rates, tiered increases, if any, and whether rates reset anytime during the year.
- To guarantee insurance payments, remind clients who haven't done so to complete initial authorization requests and call you back with certification information; to prevent future surprises, advise clients of any limits to their services, reassuring them that you will help them to secure continued care.

Referrals

In situations in which clients have no insurance benefits or their benefits have already run out, you can review choices they have for affordable care. You could offer a self-pay option; for clients in significant financial distress you could also provide a sliding fee scale (see pages 83–85). If benefits have been exhausted and you are contracted with clients' insurance carriers to accept a discounted rate, you can offer continued care to financially disadvantaged clients at the same lower rate. Many insurance companies require this regardless of clients' financial status, stipulating in their provider agreements that you cannot collect more than your contracted rate when providing services to subscribers, even when treatment extends beyond benefit limits. For people who are not in crisis or in need of weekly sessions, you could also suggest spreading out visits to make services affordable.

If none of these options work out, you can offer clients two or more low and/or no cost referrals (see pages 77–78, 83). You can also say, "If any of these referrals do not work out or you need more assistance, feel free to call me and I will be happy to help you." It can be very frustrating after people finally get the courage to ask for help, to then run into delays in getting what they need. This can happen when referral numbers are no longer in service, therapists are on vacation, schedules are booked, calls are not returned, or any number of other problems arise. By offering yourself as a back-up resource, you convey caring and stability, and, when needed, help clients again to connect to services. Even small gestures like these can benefit your practice, too; people will remember your efforts and let others know, building your positive reputation and increasing the chances of future referrals to you.

Reminders

If you are reviewing benefits over the phone, before ending calls remind clients again of their first appointment details. Although this may seem redundant and unnecessary, keep in mind that new clients are often acutely distressed before beginning therapy. They could be so anxious, depressed, or otherwise compromised that remembering payment information—much less getting to initial sessions—may be a monumental effort. Every reminder can help them get to your office at the right time and with the correct payment in hand (see pages 96–97).

Issue	Recommendation
Providing service options and reminders before the client's first session.	1) To provide services for clients with no insurance benefits, present alternative payment and referral options, offering yourself as a back-up resource if needed (p. 120). 2) To assist clients in remembering their payment details, review them before ending calls, even when you have already done so before (pp. 96–97).

CHAPTER SIX

Billing Insurance Carriers and Getting Paid Quickly

If you work with insured clients and accept payment directly from their insurance carriers, you can streamline this process by setting up your own low-maintenance insurance billing system. Clients will be relieved and appreciative to learn that you are handling this potentially stressful task. By following the steps described in this chapter to routinely bill for services, you can keep billing costs low and receipts high with minimal effort. You will read about billing using manual systems, computer software programs, online clearinghouse services, and insurance company websites. Additionally, you will learn how to streamline your routine to efficiently complete billing by the end of your work week. Simple strategies will also help you monitor outstanding claims and quickly correct common payment mistakes and denials to ensure a steady income stream.

Electronic Billing Trend

As you consider what billing method works best for your practice, be aware that there is a predicted trend away from paper claims and toward electronic billing. An article in the September 2003 *American Psychological Association* (APA) *Monitor*, titled "The Drive for Electronic Claims," describes a major reason behind this shift: the Health Insurance Portability and

Accountability Act (HIPAA) Transaction Rule, which became effective on October 16, 2003. This law aims to create national standards for the electronic transmission of health information.

The good news for now is that if you submit paper claims you are exempt from these transaction requirements. However, the law also allows insurance companies to require participating providers to submit claims electronically. At the time of this writing, the Centers for Medicare and Medicaid Services (CMS) requires electronic billing, but exempts solo practitioners and groups with ten or fewer full-time employees. The APA Practice Organization anticipates that in time many insurance companies will require filing of electronic claims. If so, carriers may follow CMS and allow individual and small group practitioners to continue submitting paper claims. Or, they could exercise their option to require everyone to file electronically.

Now you can use any billing option in your private practice. However, to be prepared in case electronic billing is required in the future, I'd recommend choosing a computer software billing system with electronic billing capability. Then, you can set up electronic billing right away or defer online billing until you are comfortable using the billing program for paper claims. Or, you can continue doing paper billing and wait to see if electronic billing is mandated later. Whatever happens, you will be able to continue billing using your computer system, ensuring that your claims are paid.

Become HIPAA Compliant

Before you start billing for your services, make sure you are in compliance with all current HIPAA laws. In addition to standardizing transmission of electronic information, HIPAA protects confidentiality and access to this data through privacy and security rules. Initially, securing compliance may seem to require an overwhelming array of new tasks. However, many are steps that clinicians routinely take in the course of everyday practice, such as securing client records and requiring written releases. HIPAA formalizes many of these tasks by mandating policies and procedures, postings in your office, and forms for clients to sign.

Technically you may not be required to become HIPAA compliant if you do not bill electronically for your services. However, penalties for non-compliance can be severe and situations outside your control could automatically trigger compliance requirements. For example, if you choose a billing or clearinghouse service that submits claims electronically, both you and the service must follow HIPAA laws. Your professional associations and publications are a good place to find workshops and materials that offer current information, steps to take, and forms you need for HIPAA compliance.

In addition to required HIPAA forms, make sure clients read, complete, and sign an informed consent form at their first session. This document informs clients of your professional services and business policies. Although you can individualize it for your practice, important areas to cover are a description of your services, fees, billing and cancellation policies, confidentiality limits, emergency procedures, release of information, and consent to treatment. Your professional associations and publications can provide details and sample agreements to use when creating your consent form.

For example, the following is a typical billing policy

> Upon verification of health plan/insurance coverage and policy limits, your insurance carrier will be billed for you and your provider will be paid directly by the carrier. You are responsible for paying any applicable deductibles and co-payments at the time services are rendered. If you are not eligible at the time services are rendered, you are responsible for full payment.

A related release of information reads:

> I authorize the release of information regarding my care to the health plan for the payment of claims, certification/case management decisions, and other purposes related to the administration of benefits for my health plan.

For efficiency, you can combine this consent form with individual and insurance intake questions. To help create your own form, an example of a combined form is included in Appendix D.

Billing Options

You have several billing options to consider for your practice. They include hiring a billing service or doing billing yourself using computer or manual systems.

Billing Service

If you absolutely do not want to do billing yourself, you can hire an outside billing service or pay an individual to do this task. However, you will pay a substantial expense for this service, usually between 7 and 10 percent of collected receipts from a billing service, or an hourly fee or salary for office help. If you are getting started in practice or planning for a part-time clientele (e.g., four to ten clients), a reasonable estimate of such an expense would be $200 a month. If you have full-time hours (e.g., twenty-five to thirty clients), fees could climb to $800 a month or higher. Keep in mind that this expense is in addition to other costs such as office rent, supplies, and continuing education workshops.

You may be thinking that it's still worth the cost to hire a billing specialist to take care of these unpleasant details. If you are constantly disorganized and procrastinate when it comes to doing routine tasks, it may be. You may relish the idea of someone else taking care of billing details, assuming that by paying a fee everything will get taken care of. But consider that not all billing services will go to the extra effort to make sure you get paid. They may accept denials or not aggressively pursue unpaid claims, especially if your collections and, in turn, their payments, will be small compared to other higher volume billing clients.

A few months into my first practice experience, Nancy, a colleague who had joined the same large group practice, came to me with a long computer printout from the group's billing service in her hand. She could not make sense of the information, as there were many shorthand terms and it was hard to identify her billed services and accompanying receipts. Upon joining the group, we were assured that our group contract provided for an outside company to handle all billing and collections for insured services. However, to assist the company in fulfilling these tasks, we were responsible for recording and sending weekly service logs to the billing service. These logs took time and effort, as we were required to write down each service we provided along with identifying information, such as the client's name, CPT code, and the date of service.

I looked at Nancy's printout and was also confused by the entries, but one thing I immediately saw was that her past few monthly payments were nowhere near the amount that she had billed. Even with insurance discounts factored in, something was very wrong. I encouraged Nancy to talk with the billing contact, and after a few attempts to reach the specialist, she was finally able to sit down in person and review the printout.

She learned that some insurance companies had denied services for various reasons, and the billing agent was uncertain what action to take to correct the problems. Other insurance providers had not yet responded to bills and again the agent was not sure why. Some clients had not responded to initial mailed bills and also owed outstanding fees. The agent assured her that all outstanding payments would be pursued, and within a month or two Nancy did receive some of her hard earned money. She also began reviewing each new billing printout in detail, calling the billing agent regularly to ensure that she would be paid for her services. However, when I left the group a couple of months later, Nancy still hadn't received a large portion of long overdue payments, totaling over a thousand dollars.

While at this large group practice, I also monitored billing service printouts and payments for my services, frequently contacting the billing agent to facilitate payments. I suspect the only reason I did not suffer the losses that Nancy did was that I had asked about billing discrepancies after receiving my first printout and continually each month that I worked in the group. This took time, effort, and seemed like a duplication of services. It was frustrating to pay for a service where I had to first record and send information to the billing service and then later doublecheck everything to be sure that I was appropriately reimbursed.

Selecting a Billing Service

Although not everyone who hires a billing service will experience what Nancy and I did, losses can happen more often than you think and when you least expect them. If you do decide to hire a billing service, ask for strong personal references from your colleagues and professional organizations. Call three or more companies and inquire about their practices and rates. Choose one that offers the option of electronic billing, specializes in mental health claims, has a clientele of private practitioners, is experienced in dealing with managed care insurance, has been in business a while (e.g., five years or longer), and provides a billing agent who is easily accessible during business hours.

If possible, visit the service and personally meet with your billing agent. Observe whether he or she interacts in a professional manner, is responsive to questions, and explains information in understandable terms. Ask to be shown how records are kept, making sure they are all secure and locked, including hard copies and computer files. Look at a sample billing printout and make sure you can understand all identifiers and clearly read your billed amounts and payments. Confirm that the service is compliant with the latest HIPAA laws and cooperative with any steps you are mandated by HIPAA to take, such as a written business associate contract.

Manual Billing

If you decide to do your own billing, you can eliminate the cost of an outside billing service or office manager and retain complete control over your earnings. Once you learn the basics, you can routinely finish this task quickly with minimal effort. If you do not like computers, do not have one, or for any other reason do not want to use a computer billing program, you can even do billing by hand or using a typewriter if you prefer. This option may be desirable if you plan on having a very small clientele and/or see just a few clients with insurance.

To save time, fill out a CMS (HCFA)-1500 claim form for each client (a UB-92 claim form for in-patient clients), which includes almost all client information except details of future services you will provide. Most insurance companies accept this standard claim form, and by asking during routine benefit checks, you will discover the occasional carrier that does not. In these rare cases, create a separate master claim using that company's required form. Then, copy these forms and fill in the dates, procedure codes, authorization numbers (if required), charges, and your signature each time you bill a client's insurance carrier. You'll just need to be sure your insurance providers accept photocopied claim forms; some use a computer scanning technology and will only recognize the red ink on original CMS (HCFA)-1500 claims. All you need for this simple billing system is CMS (HCFA)-1500 claim forms—which you can find in most office/medical supply stores—envelopes and stamps.

One-Write Ledger Systems

I started out using a manual billing method, typing master claim forms for each client, copying them, and filling in service information for each bill. I also used a manual "one-write" pegboard ledger system to record services provided to each client, charges, and payments collected. I learned about this system from my colleague Denise, who had been using it for years. If you do not want to use a computer for these practice management tasks, this is a low-cost, efficient alternative. It worked well for me regardless of my practice size—when I started out seeing fewer than ten clients and also when I was scheduling twenty-five to thirty sessions weekly.

The one-write system is designed so clients' individual ledger cards, which contain a record of services for a particular client, fit over daily log forms; when you record services provided you only write it once and it is automatically copied on your daily log. The log provides a daily, weekly, and monthly overview of your services and receipts, and the ledger cards detail this information for each client. By referring to your entries on clients' ledger cards, you can determine what services need to be billed and monitor payments. These systems also provide a business checkbook version, where you can write checks manually and automatically copy the information in a disbursements journal. If these low-tech options are of interest, you can find them in office supply stores or by doing an Internet search using the phrase *one-write systems*.

Issue	Recommendation
Choosing a billing method for your practice.	1) To be prepared in case electronic billing is required in the future, choose a computer software billing system with both paper and electronic billing capabilities (pp. 122–123). 2) To protect client information, become HIPAA compliant; to inform clients of your services and policies, provide a consent form at the first session (pp. 123–124). 3) To avoid expensive fees and doublechecking receipts for accuracy, consider doing billing yourself (pp. 125–126). 4) If you do hire a billing service, for maximum quality and accuracy, obtain personal references and compare companies' practices and rates (pp. 126–127). 5) For streamlined manual billing, prepare master claim forms for each client; to efficiently record services, use a one-write pegboard ledger system (pp. 127–128).

Computer Billing

I recommend computer billing programs as the most cost-effective, time-saving method to streamline billing and practice management tasks. You may be concerned that you are not technologically savvy and that the entire process sounds complicated and overwhelming. Investigate a bit and you may be surprised how simple computer billing can be. Computer billing/practice management programs have become very user friendly and you can selectively use only the features necessary to meet your practice needs. With careful shopping, you can keep costs low and similar to other practice items, you can claim program expenditures as a tax-deductible business expense.

Benefits

Whether your practice is small or large, a computer program will automate billing efficiently and keep track of client and insurance information, claim status, authorizations, payments, etc. Some programs also offer the feature of automatically processing credit card payments. You can also generate a variety of reports to help manage your practice. For example, an outstanding insurance report allows you to track services you have billed that have not yet been paid. This is a report I use frequently in my practice; I find it very helpful in identifying and facilitating unpaid claims. A client by referral source report details where your referrals are coming from. A log report provides a weekly transaction and income summary you can give to your accountant to help prepare financial statements and quarterly tax estimates. An authorization report tells you when to request future certifications. To use this billing software option, you'll just need a computer compatible with software system requirements and a printer.

Getting Started

Initially, it will take some time to become familiar with the program, set up identifiers and codes unique to your practice, and input current client and insurance data. However, after this is done, you will only need to input new client and insurance data and services you provide.

After using a manual billing system for two years, I transitioned to a computer billing/practice management system. At the time I was seeing twenty-five to thirty clients weekly and the majority had some form of insurance coverage. It took a good part of a weekend to read the manual, set the system up, and input client and insurance information. I remember making a few frustrated calls for technical support the following week as things did not go as planned for the first billing. However, after setting the system up, correcting problems in the first two or three billing cycles, and learning the routine, I was surprised at how efficiently the computerized billing program worked. I was used to writing down everything, constantly duplicating information, having to keep track of managed care authorizations, addressing envelopes, etc. Now my program saved all insurance and client information, tracked and warned me of managed care authorization limits, printed all claims on original CMS (HCFA)-1500 forms, monitored unpaid claims, and even printed envelope mailing labels for each insurance carrier. The billing system continues to provide the same benefits now that my clientele is much smaller (e.g., eight to twelve clients weekly).

Selecting a Billing/Practice Management Program

You can learn of helpful billing/practice management programs through your colleagues, professional advertisements, and organizations. A simple way to start your search is to survey two or three colleagues who do their own computer billing to find out what software they are using. Ask what they like and don't like about the product and whether they would choose it again. Most professional newsletters, magazines, and journals also contain software advertisements in every issue. You could call your local or national organization (e.g., APA, NASW) for suggestions or search their websites; they may have a current listing of programs, comparing features and prices of each. You can also find programs by doing an Internet search for "mental health billing and practice management software."

Before choosing, call two or more companies to compare their software products and costs, which can vary by hundreds and even thousands of dollars. Some offer one package and others charge additional fees for different features, which can add up quickly. You may not even use many of these separately priced options (e.g., case management, treatment plans, progress notes, and scheduling), so for the best savings don't pay for more than you need. Confirm that the companies you are considering offer software with electronic billing capability. Look for a company that has been in business a while (e.g., five years or more), whose software is designed for individual or small group mental health practices versus large agencies, and is compliant with current HIPAA laws.

Upgrades and Technical Support

Companies vary widely on policies and pricing for upgrades and technical support. Some require that you pay for yearly program updates and support contracts. This can be quite costly. For the most savings, look for companies that offer optional upgrades and ongoing technical support at no cost or for a reasonable one-time fee. Once you set up your program and do some billing runs, you may not need frequent upgrades or technical support. By paying for these features only when needed, you can save hundreds when you're getting started in practice and thousands over years of your practice.

My colleague, Megan, bought her computer billing program years ago before Windows was developed, when DOS was the standard operating system. She chose a company with complimentary technical support and optional, reasonably priced updates. After setting up her system there were few problems and she rarely needed to call technical support. Although updates were regularly offered, she opted not to buy them since her program fulfilled all her billing needs.

However, when computer systems changed from DOS to Windows, she decided it was time to buy a new computer with a Windows operating system. After transferring her DOS-based billing program to the new computer, she bought the Windows upgrade and was able to transfer all her data to the faster, updated program. Since then, she has not needed or purchased another upgrade, and in many years of practice has saved thousands of dollars because she was not required to buy yearly updates or support contracts.

When comparing software choices, speak with someone in the company's technical support and see whether he or she is helpful, respectful, patient, and knowledgeable in responding to your questions. Check whether answers are clear and understandable. Ask for the tech support hours during the week and weekend. Consider choosing a company located as close to your time zone as possible, so when you need to call for support, a technician is likely to be available. Most companies allow you to sample their programs before buying, either at no cost or for a small fee that you may be able to apply toward the cost of the program. Once you narrow down your choices to two or three programs, try out each option to see which one you prefer.

When I chose my billing software I didn't give any thought to where the company and technicians were located. I was just pleased to learn that technical support was available by phone on Fridays and Saturdays, days I planned for billing and learning the software program. What I soon discovered was that around the time I ran into problems with the billing program it was early afternoon for me on the West Coast and almost quitting time for the technicians on the East Coast. Although I was usually able to get my questions answered in time, it would have been much less stressful if the technicians were in the same time zone, especially in the beginning when I was setting up the program.

You'll find that the time and effort you put in now to research companies and choose your software program will be well worth it in the long run. Selecting a stable, well-run company and affordable program is important because it's in your best interest to stay with the same billing program for the life of your practice. Although you can always switch software, it will take time and effort to learn a new system and input client and insurance information. If you have been in practice for a while, you will probably not want the extra workload of manually transferring years of old data to a new program. The downside of keeping old data on an obsolete program is that you will have to refer back to the old program anytime you want to reference previous information.

Issue	Recommendation
Choosing and setting up a computer software billing system.	1) For the most efficient and cost-effective billing, choose a computer software billing system (pp. 128–129). 2) To transition to a computer billing system, set aside time (e.g., a weekend) to install and learn the program, enlisting outside aid as needed (pp. 129–130). 3) To find billing/practice management programs, survey colleagues, professional advertisements, and organizations (p. 130). 4) To choose an affordable, high-quality program, buy one specializing in mental health, with e-billing capability, and that offers optional upgrades and reasonable fee-for-service technical support (pp. 130–131). 5) To choose software with optimum technical support, compare technicians at each company, ideally located in your time zone; to select a program you prefer, sample software finalists before deciding on one (pp. 131–132).

Electronic Billing

Another billing option is to send claims electronically to a clearinghouse, which modifies and sends them on to individual insurance companies. Although some billing services offer online billing, your best choice is to use a computer software billing program configured for electronic billing.

In addition to a computer and billing software, you typically need a modem, transmission line, and in most cases Internet access, which you may already have. To protect your computer from destructive viruses and privacy intrusions, install a virus protection program and firewall on your computer before sending any electronic claims. These are available in any computer/office supply store and are well worth the initial cost and yearly update fees. Most antivirus or firewall programs offer the feature of automatically updating protection, or you can perform the update manually, preferably weekly.

Select a Program with Electronic Billing Capability

Even if you don't plan to do electronic billing, compare e-billing options of billing software programs before choosing one so you will be prepared in case this billing method is required in the future. You can find e-billing information on the websites of billing software companies, on their demo programs, and by calling their sales and technical support. Note the names of the clearinghouses affiliated with each software choice, their contact numbers, and how long they have been in business. Compare pricing, which usually includes a one-time set-up fee, recurring charge per claim, and sometimes an additional monthly service fee.

Clearinghouses may limit transmittals to certain insurance companies, so look for one that can send and receive claims to the insurance companies you plan to bill. Talk with a technician at each clearinghouse and compare how available, helpful, and responsive they are to your questions. Verify that each clearinghouse is HIPAA compliant.

Deferring Electronic Billing

If you will be using a computer software billing system for the first time, it will be easier to defer electronic billing until you become familiar with and comfortable generating paper claims. Especially if you have limited time and/or view this task as aversive, you'll be able to set up e-billing faster when you don't have the added work of setting up computer billing at the same time.

Before switching to electronic billing, be aware that it is continually evolving. In recent years, submission requirements and billing formats have undergone many changes. With the passage of HIPAA laws, these modifications are likely to continue in the foreseeable future. And based on past experience, clearinghouses that are viable now may not be in the future. You could go to all the work and expense of setting up electronic billing through a clearinghouse only to find out later that the company is going out of business.

I can confirm from my own frustrating experience that this does happen. After years of printing paper claims, I decided to try electronic billing offered by my software billing company through a well-known clearinghouse. Since my software was already configured for e-billing, I just needed to input electronic codes for insurance companies and install the clearinghouse communications software. I was very excited about the proposed benefits; no more work of printing claims and mailing labels, no more sorting through papers and stuffing envelopes, and each claim cost less than the price of a stamp.

After spending time setting up the system and calling the clearinghouse technician to correct problems in the first few billing runs, I was very pleased with the outcome. The clearinghouse was able to electronically transmit bills to all of the insurance companies I worked with, and soon I was receiving payments two to three weeks faster than I ever did with paper claims. All I had to do to send claims to the clearinghouse was to type a few commands on the computer.

All was going very smoothly until a few months later when I made a routine call to technical support with a question about a claim. I was told that technicians were not available and when I asked why, I heard the shocking news. The clearinghouse was going out of business very soon and was in the process of phasing out technical support. There were no plans to reorganize or merge with another company, so in a short time my elec-tronic software would be unusable. This news hit hard. After taking the time and effort to set up this system, learn the protocol to transmit claims, and ensure successful billings, everything changed in one phone call.

Fortunately, after the clearinghouse closed down, my billing software could still generate paper claims, and I have continued using this method of billing ever since. Although my software program has now affiliated with new clearinghouses, I am hesitant to do e-billing again, acutely aware of how quickly companies can come and go in this ever-changing high-tech environment. However, if electronic billing becomes mandatory, my program is capable of connecting to a clearinghouse for e-billing if needed.

Insurance Website Billing

Some insurance companies offer the option of billing directly through their websites. By obtaining a user ID and password you can go to their websites, type in patient identifying information and services provided, receive payment, and check on claim status. Some companies offer this at no cost and others charge a fee for the software required to connect to their system. Especially for carriers that offer billing at no cost, this option may sound great. You don't have to do manual or paper billing or even bother with electronic clearinghouses. By logging onto a website and typing some information for each claim, you can get payment quickly with little effort or expense.

Although this option may initially sound optimal, it's likely that not every insurance company you work with will offer this billing option. Those that do will each have different requirements and protocols. You will have the job of logging onto multiple websites, generating bills at each one, and constantly jumping back and forth between them to keep track of payments, outstanding claims, and to correct errors. And for insurance carriers that do not offer website billing, you'll have to use a different method altogether to bill those companies. If you use a manual or computer billing system to record services and generate claims, you'll want to document all of the services you provide, including those you bill through websites. Therefore, you will end up recording your services in two places, duplicating work that you could complete by using just your manual or computer billing system alone.

Given these problems, website billing is the most feasible if you have a small number of insured clients covered through one or two companies that offer website billing. You'll just have a couple of websites to keep track of and you won't have too many services to record twice. For example, my friend Dawn has a small practice with mostly self-pay clients. Her remaining clientele is exclusively insured through the one managed care company Dawn is contracted with as a preferred provider. She collects fees from her self-pay clients at the time of their sessions and bills the insurance company through the provider website for remaining services. She has just one website to keep track of, records the insurance services a second time in her manual log book, and benefits from the rapid payments she receives from the managed care company.

Issue	Recommendation
Considering options of electronic and insurance website billing.	1) To find electronic billing clearinghouses, survey software billing company websites, their demo programs, and/or each company's sales/technical support staff (pp. 132–133). 2) To choose an affordable, high-quality clearinghouse for electronic billing, compare two or more companies (p. 133). 3) To reduce work overload when setting up a computer billing system, defer electronic billing until you become comfortable generating paper claims (p. 133). 4) To avoid the problem of setting up electronic billing through a clearinghouse that may later go out of business, defer e-billing until it becomes mandatory (pp. 133–134). 5) To prevent inefficient, duplicate work, do not use website billing unless you see a small number of clients insured through one or two insurance companies (p. 135).

Streamlining Your Billing Routine

As you consider options to do billing yourself, you may be wondering how you will fit this task into your schedule along with everything else (e.g., client appointments, phone calls, verifying benefits, reports). You certainly don't want to fill your valuable free time with billing, and rightly so. After working hard in your practice you deserve a break from professional responsibilities. And by preserving time to recharge your batteries you'll be better able to serve your clients and maintain your health. With this time factor in mind, building steps efficiently into your routine will allow you to do a little each day to finish billing by the end of your work week. The following protocol describes procedures to ensure timely billing and a steady income flow without cutting into your personal time. Although the focus is on using a computer system for paper billing, suggestions will also apply if you send claims electronically or use a manual billing system.

Take Your Computer to Work

The first component essential to your routine is to always have your computer billing system at work when you are seeing clients. When your system is readily available, you can use time between sessions and during unscheduled hours for billing and related practice management tasks, such as inputting client, insurance, and service data, typing progress notes, and completing reports. If you work full-time in one office that is very secure, you may prefer a desktop computer. However, if you want access to your computer at home and/or you work part-time in one or more locations, I recommend a laptop computer.

Use a Laptop Computer

Every year as technology advances, laptops become lighter, more powerful, and less expensive. They are easy to carry and use wherever you are—at home, at your office(s), when traveling, etc. You can power it with included components of an adaptor or battery if an outlet is not available. All information is in one place and by keeping it with you at all times you can preserve confidentiality of information and protect it from theft. And. you will have complete flexibility to do billing and other tasks wherever and whenever you want. You'll just need to be sure your portable computer is secure at all times, as lightweight laptops are easier to misplace and steal compared to bulkier desktops.

A fellow clinician named Frank sublets office space in two nearby cities. He spends two days a week in each city and has a general psychotherapy practice that includes couples, families, and children. Due to their work and school schedules, a majority of his clients come to sessions after 3 P.M. Many days Frank ends up with unscheduled appointment hours in the morning or early afternoon, time he could use for billing and practice management tasks. The only obstacle preventing him from using this time is that he does not have his computer system at the office. He has a desktop model, which he keeps at home and uses on Fridays, the day he has set aside to complete practice tasks. To utilize his desktop at work he would have to move it back and forth between home and each office daily, which would be cumbersome and time consuming. Although he could leave the computer in each office overnight, he does not feel comfortable risking confidentiality violations and theft.

If Frank switched to a laptop computer he could easily take it with him to each office and use available hours and minutes between sessions for billing tasks. By using work time efficiently, by the end of his client week he could potentially finish billing and other practice chores, freeing Fridays and weekends to do whatever he wants. If he falls behind, he could use Friday to catch up and still preserve his weekends. He likes the idea of having more free time to pursue his new passion, golf, and plans to buy a laptop to facilitate this goal.

Set Up Your Printer(s)

If you want the ability to print information at more than one location, you could buy a printer (or a printer/copier/fax machine all-in-one) and connecting cable for each primary place you'll be (e.g., home, office[s]). Although most printers are less portable than laptop computers, they have become inexpensive and are well worth the small investment. For example, if you sublet office space, you could keep a printer in the office(s) and one at home, giving you the flexibility to print claims, client notes, reports, and other information at either location.

Bill Weekly

Once you have your computer and printer(s) in place, the next step is to establish a daily routine for tasks you'll need to complete in order to generate and send insurance claims at the end of the week. Although you can bill at any interval you want, I'd recommend billing weekly. This keeps your task small, consistent, and manageable compared to accumulating a month or more backlog of unrecorded and unbilled services. By billing frequently you will also generate a steady income flow. You will receive payment denials or mistakes sooner, giving you the chance to fix them and get paid for your services as soon as possible.

Note that most insurance companies have deadlines for submitting bills after providing services (e.g., sixty to ninety days). The last thing you need is to fall behind in billing and be denied payment for services because you missed the deadline to submit claims. Weekly billing will prevent this from happening, and you'll never have the stress of racing around at the last minute to beat the clock when submitting your claims.

Back Up Your Data

Another important task to build in weekly is to externally back up your billing program data and other practice management files. If you have a large practice and enter a high volume of new data frequently to your program, you may prefer to conduct daily backups. This will protect crucial information if your hard drive crashes, saving much time and stress when restoring your program.

Your billing program manual or technical support can recommend optimal backup methods for your system. For example, your computer may have a built-in CD burner (CD-RW drive) you can use, or you could buy an external CD-RW drive at a reasonable cost. Other options are a DVD burner (DVD-RW drive), zip drive, flash drive, external hard drive, or tape backup system. All of these choices are available at computer/office supply stores. You can also backup data to 3½ inch floppy disks, but this method can be time-consuming and require many disks, especially as your data files grow larger the longer you are in practice.

When conducting a backup, alternate between three or more backup mediums to avoid the problem of unreadable data, which can happen when just one or two backup sets are overused. To safeguard your data, always keep a current backup in a separate location. For example, if you keep a backup at home and at the office and a fire destroys your home, you can use your office backup and avoid a second tragedy of losing all your data.

Schedule Forty-five Minute Sessions

To create a manageable daily routine, as soon as you get to the office, turn on your computer and leave it on throughout your workday. You will then be able to quickly use it between sessions without wasting time turning it on and off. If you're using a laptop, plug it into an outlet to prevent wearing down the battery. When scheduling clients, consider offering forty-five- as opposed to fifty-minute appointments, and end sessions on time. This will give you five extra minutes to complete client-oriented and billing tasks between sessions. It may not seem like much, but fifteen minutes can go a long way toward getting tasks done, especially when you develop a habitual routine.

Issue	Recommendation
Taking initial steps to set up a streamlined billing routine.	1) To ensure a steady income flow and preserve your personal time, set up a daily and weekly billing routine (p. 136). 2) To efficiently use time at work for billing, have your computer system readily accessible at the office; for maximum portability, use a laptop instead of a desktop computer (pp. 137–138). 3) For the ability to print information at any time, buy an inexpensive printer for each work location (p. 138). 4) To keep claims manageable, correct payment mistakes quickly, and beat submission deadlines, set up billing at the end of every week (p. 138). 5) To protect billing data, conduct weekly backups, keeping one set in a separate location; to allow time between sessions for billing tasks, offer forty-five-minute appointments and end sessions on time (p. 139).

Completing Billing and Office Tasks Between Sessions

Several steps will help you complete billing and office tasks during your work week. They include attending to client-oriented tasks, recording your services and payments, using unexpected time at work and scheduling daily and weekly time to finish tasks.

Client-Oriented Tasks

Between sessions, attend to clients' needs before anything else. Check for new messages and return client inquiries and urgent calls right away. Then type client progress notes for the previous session, which will be easier when the details are fresh in your mind. By completing them between sessions during your day, you will also prevent a large backlog of unfinished notes. Your progress notes will be better too when you only have to focus on typing one at a time. For the sake of efficiency, use a word processing program, which usually comes standard on any computer you buy. You will then be able to move back and forth between your billing and word processing programs, quickly completing practice management tasks. After finishing your progress note, prepare for the next client session (review progress notes and treatment plans, organize interventions, etc).

These client-oriented tasks may already seem to easily fill up fifteen minutes, but keep in mind that you will not have client inquiry or urgent calls waiting for you to return between every session. Unless you type very long notes or need to document details from a complicated session, your progress note will require only a couple of minutes or so. Your pre-session review will also go faster as you become familiar with ongoing clients and remember details about their treatment more quickly. And, by using an automated computer billing system, you won't need much additional time to complete the following billing tasks.

Recording Your Service

During remaining minutes between sessions, go into your billing program to record the session you just finished. For ongoing clients, you will have already created a file for each person that includes, among other things, personal and insurance information, authorization details, and identifiers for claim forms. For these established clients, open their files to record the service you just provided. Many programs call this a ledger entry, which typically includes the date of service, diagnosis, CPT code, insurance carrier and client fees, authorization, if needed, and special notes you wish to add. Each entry is automatically recorded and saved in individual client ledgers and a central daily log. Many programs have a feature that lets you copy your previous ledger entry to create a new one, saving the time and work of typing duplicate information week after week when providing the same service regularly to clients.

Recording the Client's Payment

After recording your service, add any payment collected from your client during the session. This creates another ledger/daily log entry, and typically includes the client name, amount paid, check number or cash, and the applicable service date. Once you've entered service and payment information, you're done recording that session. These two steps combined should take less than five minutes; as you get used to the routine you can go faster. The key is to complete entries between sessions, breaking the seemingly huge billing project down into small tasks that fit into your day.

Preventing a Backlog of Unfinished Work

As you read about completing these between-session tasks, you may be concerned that unexpected events could easily put you behind, creating a stressful backlog of unfinished work. Perhaps a prospective client calls you in crisis after being diagnosed with cancer, needing extra time and help to stabilize during the inquiry call. Or, your child calls from home because he misses you and is upset after fighting with a friend at school. Maybe your office neighbor and friend stops by for a casual talk, and you'd like to catch up on things since you haven't seen her in a while. These and other situations can and do happen at any time, often when you least expect them. You can count on the fact that some days will not go as planned and your pile of unfinished tasks will start to grow.

On days when you do get behind, you can still prevent unfinished work from snowballing into a massive, unmanageable monster. The sooner you clean up the backlog, the easier it will be to get back to your routine. Just as you encounter time-draining events, you will also gain unanticipated minutes and hours when clients arrive late for appointments or do not show. With your computer readily available, you can efficiently use this otherwise wasted time to finish these tasks. New client files may also take more time to enter than you will have between sessions. For these first-time clients, you can defer creating files and entering services until a non-scheduled hour or right after your last client that day.

Scheduling Daily Time for Tasks

On any given day you'll probably end up with one or more unscheduled work hours to use; you can also actively schedule your day to ensure available time. For example, you could arrive at work an hour before seeing your first client and/or leave an hour after finishing with your last client of the day. Or, if you work mornings, leave in the afternoons to pick up your children from school and return for evening clients when your spouse is home—you could schedule an extra hour in the morning and/or evening for these tasks.

One of my former office neighbors, Joan, a clinician in full-time practice for over ten years, decided to enroll in a psychoanalytic training program. Her seminars began at 7:30 P.M. Tuesday and Thursday nights, and I often saw her through my office window rushing out of the building after her 6 p.m. client. The training institute was about a forty-five minute drive from the office, depending on traffic, and Joan remarked that sometimes she would arrive late for the lecture, much to her dismay. She also noticed that tasks she was usually able to finish on Tuesday after her 6 p.m. client were put off until Wednesday, and so on until Friday. Soon she fell a week behind and then two, until eventually tasks were months overdue. Her insurance payments slowed while her stress accelerated, and when she started to feel sick she realized something had to give.

Since Joan was committed to the program and classes were always at the same time, she decided to end her last client sessions on Tuesdays and Thursdays at 6 P.M. instead of 7 P.M. As soon as she added the extra hour to her days, she was able to finish daily chores before leaving the office, and eventually caught up on the backlog of work. Instead of rushing around at the last minute on class days, Joan was now able to get everything done and leave early, making sure she got to class in time to hear every lecture.

Recording Insurance Payments

By using scheduled and unscheduled time during your workday, you can often complete daily billing tasks by the time you go home. One additional billing job you'll have is to record insurance payments. About a month or so after you start sending paper claims weekly, you'll generate a stream of incoming checks from insurance carriers. Record these reimbursements by going into your computer billing program and crediting corresponding client files. Each credit creates an additional ledger/daily log entry, which usually includes the client and insurance name, the amount paid, the check number, and the applicable date of service. As claims problems will arise, you'll need to call insurance carriers to correct errors when they occur.

Finishing Progress Notes and Other Duties

You can also use any extra time for other duties such as creating client files, calling insurance carriers for benefit checks, returning non-client calls, reading mail and professional publications, typing reports/correspondence, consulting with colleagues, purchasing supplies, and paying bills. And by taking a couple of steps, you can quickly finish your progress notes. After typing notes for the day, print and place them in each client's file. For easy transfer to client files, print them on full-page, "quick peel" transcription sheets, which you can find in office supply stores. Starting with the first note at the top of the transcription sheet, cut out each one, peel off the back, and affix it to a blank paper sheet in each client's file.

Completing Authorizations

One final activity you'll need time for is authorizations. If you work with managed care insurance companies, you will need to complete treatment requests and record new authorizations you receive. Most billing programs are able to record and track authorizations, alerting you when limits are reached. After receiving new authorizations, enter the details in each client's file, including the certification number, services and total sessions approved, and the timeframe in which the client can use them.

Scheduling Weekly Backup Time to Finish Tasks

If all goes as planned and you complete billing tasks each day, by the end of the week all you'll have left to complete billing is to close your daily log, print insurance claims and mailing labels, sign claims, and drop them in the mail. To bypass the tedious task of signing each claim, you can use a signature stamp instead, which most office supply stores can create using a sample of your signature. However, as I said earlier, even when using all available time, you may not always get every task done daily that you planned. More than likely, you will have days when things get put off until the next day or longer.

To provide a backup if you fall behind, schedule a large block of time at the end of your client week to finish billing and other practice management tasks. Similar to Frank, many clinicians schedule clients Monday through Thursday, keeping Friday open for billing and other professional/personal activities. The amount of time to schedule will depend on the size of your practice, how many insured clients you have, and how much you get done during the week. To provide ample time for the weeks you fall very behind, it's best to always reserve more as opposed to less time (e.g., one day versus one-half day, four versus two hours). If you do get everything done before the end of your scheduled backup time, you can stop early and take advantage of additional free time.

Facilitating Insurance Payments

Several practices will help you facilitate insurance payments. These include generating outstanding claims reports, calling insurance carriers about unpaid bills, recording your contacts, dealing with missing and incorrect claims, and engaging supervisors and select clients for assistance.

Issue	Recommendation
Completing billing and other practice management tasks during your work week.	1) To ensure priority client needs are addressed, between sessions first complete client-oriented tasks before anything else (pp. 140–141). 2) To efficiently record the previous session in your computer billing program, enter the service you just provided and any client payment you received (p. 141). 3) To prevent a stressful backlog of unfinished work, use time when clients come late or do not show to complete tasks, and/or schedule your day to ensure available time (pp. 141–143). 4) To finish practice tasks, create new client files, record insurance payments/authorizations, file progress notes, and print/send insurance claims (pp. 143–144). 5) To provide backup time to complete unfinished tasks, schedule a block of time at the end of your client week (p. 144).

Outstanding Claims Reports

By conducting insurance benefit checks before initial sessions, you can greatly reduce the likelihood of problems in receiving insurance payments for your services. However, occasionally you may still encounter road-blocks to getting paid. For various reasons insurance carriers can get behind in payments, pay incorrect amounts, and sometimes not send payments at all. To facilitate timely payment and assist in correcting payment mistakes, six weeks after sending paper claims, generate and print an outstanding insurance report using your computer billing program. Create these reports routinely—biweekly or monthly. Each report shows all services that were billed before a designated date (e.g., six weeks ago) and have not yet been paid. Information typically includes service dates, amounts due, patient identifiers, insurance names, and claim contact numbers.

Calling Insurance Carriers

For each unpaid service listed on your report, call the matching insurance carrier to find out why. Choose the option on their message for providers and then claims, and talk with a claims agent in person: "This is Nicole

Rogers, licensed clinical social worker, calling to facilitate payment for an outstanding claim for patient Margaret Cummings." The agent will typically ask for identifying information for you, the patient, and the date(s) of service in question.

Recording Your Contact

To accurately record your contact, write down the date you called, the agent's name, and any information you are told. By recording every contact with claims agents, you can refer to these notes to help monitor claim status and follow up later if payment is not received. For efficiency, write information on post-it notes and place them next to the corresponding service on your outstanding insurance report. Then, if needed, you can easily move these contact post-it notes to future outstanding insurance reports, avoiding the extra work of copying the information.

Missing Claims

You may learn that claims are in process but not yet completed. If so, ask the agent to estimate when you'll be paid and record the projected payment date. Another problem can occur when your claims are not received. They may have gotten lost in the mail or at any point along the way before being entered in the insurance carrier's claims database. Lost claims are by far the most common reason I encounter for unpaid services.

If your claims are missing, you can easily remedy the problem by sending a duplicate claim, which you can generate through your computer billing program. Billing a second time will delay payment another month or longer, so to speed up reimbursement, request to fax your claim to the agent for immediate processing. Also ask for an estimated payment date. Before faxing, add the following to the top of the claim: Attn: (the claims agent's name, Claims), date, the phrase "2nd submission—please expedite payment," your name, and your contact numbers.

Claims Placed on Hold

You may instead discover that your claims were received but for some reason they were not fully processed and were put on hold. This can happen when claims information is incorrect or missing (e.g., an expired or absent authorization number, an incorrect insurance address, or the wrong insured ID number). By reviewing the claim, the agent can usually identify the problem, allowing you to fix the information, and finish processing the claim.

Incorrect Payments

In other cases you will receive insurance payments that do not match what you expected to receive. Before calling to find out why, locate the client's physical file and pull out the notes from the insurance benefit check you conducted before the initial session. Refer to this information when talking with the agent to compare it to what you are told. You may learn that a claims processor made a simple mistake, such as calculating an incorrect co-payment or applying the wrong benefit level to your payment. In these cases, ask the claims agent to reprocess the claim so you won't have to submit another one. Before ending your call, ask for and add the projected payment date to your contact note.

When the information you receive does not match what you were told in the initial benefit check, the claims agent may not have the expertise or authority to adjust incorrect payments. If you get stuck trying to correct a problem, ask for a claims supervisor and explain your situation. Supervisors often have the experience and ability to fix claims problems quickly, saving you both time and frustration.

Clients as Advocates

If you still can't correct claims payments with the help of a supervisor, another option is to explain the problem to your client and ask him or her to call the insurance company. To avoid burdening your clients with potentially upsetting situations, use your clinical judgment to choose which clients to involve in claims problems. Do not engage fragile, unstable, and unassertive clients who may also resent being asked to handle this task. Instead, select assertive, stable individuals who can advocate for their benefits without emotional costs to them.

To make the call easier, give the client a copy of the insurance payment statement, called an explanation of benefits (EOB). Highlight the carrier's phone number, usually printed on the statement, and direct your client to call, selecting the option on the carrier's message recording for members and then claims. Sometimes insured clients can be the best advocates for their own benefits, especially when they are assertive and comfortable in this role.

After some frustrating calls to an insurance carrier to correct payments, I mentioned the problem to my insured client, Cherise, an assertive mother of three. I gave her a copy of the EOB and explained that services were inexplicably denied payment, and asked if she could call to request corrections. Within two weeks I received the remaining payments and when I asked Cherise what she did, she said she simply called and told the agent to pay the claims.

Claims Appeals

With most insurance companies you can also go through an appeals process to correct payment mistakes. However, this will involve more paperwork, additional time, and may still not guarantee payment. Before choosing this option, consider whether it is time- and cost-effective for you to pursue an appeal. If the outstanding insurance balance is high (e.g., hundreds of dollars), and/or you have clearly documented evidence to support your case, you may decide it's worth it to appeal. If, instead, the added stress and work outweigh the potential reimbursement, you're better off preserving your time and well-being by forgoing the appeal process altogether.

Billing/Practice Tasks Checklist

A billing/practice tasks checklist of the steps we've covered is included in Appendix E. You may wish to refer to it to help establish your own billing and practice tasks routine.

Issue	Recommendation
Facilitating insurance payments.	1) To ensure timely insurance payments, create outstanding insurance reports and call claims agents to facilitate unpaid claims (pp. 145–146). 2) To help monitor claim status and place follow-up calls when needed, record each contact you have with claims agents (p. 146). 3) To quickly process lost claims, fax them directly to claims agents; to facilitate claims placed on hold, supply missing/corrected data (p. 146). 4) To fix incorrect insurance payments, refer to benefit check information during initial calls to claims agents; enlist a supervisor's help when needed (p. 147). 5) To correct claims if other methods fail, engage select clients' help; to prevent stressful work, consider a formal appeal only if unpaid balances are high (e.g., hundreds of dollars) (pp. 147–148).

PART III
Implementing Efficient Client Policies

CHAPTER SEVEN

Managing Finances Wisely and Collecting the Fees You've Earned

In addition to weekly billing/practice tasks, you will also need to manage your receipts. This chapter helps you streamline financial tasks, walking you through weekly, monthly, and quarterly steps. You will learn efficient ways to set up a checking account, make deposits, and prepare financial reports for your practice. Tips to automate and make your tasks routine will save you time and effort.

Another essential practice task is collecting outstanding payments from clients. By collecting client fees at the time of service, you will greatly reduce how often you'll need to perform this task. However, there will be times when clients incur unexpected bills (e.g., late cancellations and no-shows). This chapter offers strategies to collect client payments while preserving therapeutic rapport. Important considerations of client factors, clinician fears, and comfort level are discussed to help implement your collections policy.

Managing Finances

Several steps will help you efficiently manage your practice finances. They include establishing business banking essentials, and preparing monthly and quarterly financial reports.

Business Banking Essentials

To establish business banking essentials, the following steps will help you set up a checking account, credit card, financial management system, checks, deposit slips, and weekly deposit routine.

Checking Account

To keep business and personal finances separate, use one bank checking account exclusively for your practice. The simplest and least expensive option is a personal (versus business) account, which will easily meet your needs as a solo practitioner. Look for an account offering the lowest minimum balance to prevent a service fee, because in private practice, your balance can periodically dip when weekly receipts are low. Also look for the lowest fees for checks you deposit that might bounce, as some clients may unexpectedly overdraw their accounts. To avoid long waits in bank lines, obtain a bankcard for convenient deposits and withdrawals at ATMs. To prepare for ATM deposits, you'll also need deposit envelopes, available at your bank or nearby ATM. To save the time and work of personally endorsing each check, order a deposit stamp from the bank, which includes your name, account number, and "For Deposit Only." Request to start your statement the first of every month so you can easily coordinate bank statements with practice management reports.

good idea

Credit Card

In addition to a checking account, obtain a separate credit card for business expenses and pay for charges through your business account. To avoid the trap of paying high-interest fees, do not charge more than you can pay off at the end of the billing cycle. For the most savings, look for a credit card with no annual fee, offering no-cost rewards such as airline miles, hotel nights, and merchandise. My colleague, Megan, has earned enough rewards for more than one domestic airline ticket by using her no-cost Visa card for business purchases and paying off her balance each month.

Financial Management System

To streamline your account activities and provide easy access to your account history, keep your business checking account on a computer software program such as Quicken (www.quicken.com). These programs are easy to use and will automatically calculate balances, reconcile your account, and offer numerous types of printable reports. You can set up categories for business expenses and income, and create monthly budget reports based on your past expenses or future projections. You can also generate financial reports to give to your accountant. And if you prefer, you can pay bills online at your convenience.

I started using Quicken over ten years ago for my business and personal checking accounts, and was immediately impressed by how helpful it was to monitor income and expenses with numeric and graphic reports. By regularly comparing expenses over the years, I identified areas to cut costs and, in turn, kept more income. For example, when reviewing one report, I realized the phone book advertisement I had been paying for in the last few years was no longer worth the monthly expense. Most new referrals were now coming from no-cost Internet insurance lists or by word of mouth, so I did not renew the ad and subsequently saved over $500 each year. I also like having rapid access to financial information. For example, I can easily avoid paying organization dues and journal subscriptions twice by searching my payment history upon receiving second bills. Often payments and second notices cross in the mail; by using the computer, I can quickly find recent payments and disregard second bills.

To provide a written backup, record transactions in your checkbook register as well as your computer program. There will be times you are away from your computer and by using your register, you can record activity to input later on the computer. Your register will also provide immediate access to your balance and activity history when your computer is not accessible. If you prefer not to use a checkbook register, write down transactions you make when away from the computer to input later.

If you prefer to record checks manually, consider a one-write system described earlier, which allows you to categorize and track weekly, monthly, and yearly expenses and deposits (see pp. 127–128). For these systems, you will need to buy matching checks that fit on top of the disbursements journal, allowing each check you write to be automatically copied on the journal underneath.

Checks

When buying checks for other systems, consider a mail-order company, whose prices are typically one-third to one-half of bank check fees. I discovered this after ordering checks from my bank for years, assuming this method was the safest and well worth the high expense. My friend, Roberta, in self-employed sales, also bought checks from her bank. After noticing that her latest check order was delayed, she realized that her account balance was mysteriously shrinking. Upon calling the bank, they surmised that her new checks must have been stolen and her account was being debited without her knowledge. Roberta had to change her account number, order new checks again, and change automatic debits from her account.

After Roberta's experience and realizing expensive bank checks are not always secure, I cautiously tried a mail-order company advertised in the Sunday paper for my next check order. I bought the four box special of duplicate, personal-sized checks, monitoring my account balance daily until the order arrived. I was pleased by how inexpensive they were and surprised at how quickly I received the order. I'm just now using my last box of checks, having saved a great deal by purchasing from an outside company.

If you have safety concerns about ordering by mail, you can contact the Better Business Bureau in advance to check the company's legitimacy and any history of complaints. You can do this quickly by logging onto the nationwide website, www.bbb.org and searching by the company's city, state, and business name.

To retain a hard copy for reference, you may prefer duplicate checks, which have slightly higher fees. However, by recording each check, you can just as easily refer to your own records. I've been using duplicate checks for years and have rarely referred to my paper copies. For my next order, I plan to save on expense and paper by choosing single checks.

Deposit Slips

Your weekly receipts may fit on the deposit slips that come standard with your checks, if so, these may work fine. If not, order the larger deposit slips, which typically have room for as many as twenty to thirty entries. Your bank may provide these at no cost upon your request.

PREPARING WEEKLY DEPOSITS. An ideal time to prepare your receipts for deposit is at the end of your client week when you are completing billing tasks. By depositing your income weekly, you will ensure a healthy account balance, preventing overdraw and penalty fees. If you use an automated billing program, you can efficiently prepare deposits when the computer is printing reports and claims. To start, fill out a deposit slip, including all income (e.g., client and insurance payments) you received that week. To retain a hard copy for future reference, photocopy the deposit slip and the individual checks you received, adding a list of cash payments by clients to your copy. Endorse the back of each check with your bank deposit stamp and place all checks, currency, and the deposit slip in an ATM bank deposit envelope. As soon as is convenient—ideally that day—go to your nearby ATM to place your deposit. If a mailbox is close to your ATM, simplify the task by making one trip to mail claims and deposit income. Record your deposit in your checkbook register and computer program.

With many activities competing for your attention, it can be easy to set your deposits aside, with good intentions to get to the ATM as soon as you get a chance. Delays can quickly expand to days and as you accumulate more mail and paperwork, your deposits can easily get buried or even thrown out with the trash. Not a happy situation to be in, as my former office mate Karen discovered. One night I walked out of my suite after a session to find Karen searching each office, the kitchen and conference rooms, the office supply area, and even the waiting room for her missing deposits. I joined the hunt, looking everywhere—under papers, on the floor, behind furniture, and in the trash—to no avail. Karen had set aside her deposits the week before, as she was busy with her normal routine plus a two-day workshop, driving her child to extra school activities, and preparing to host visitors that weekend. After a long search and no deposits, we finally stopped and Karen left in a very bad mood. As far as I know, she never did find those receipts, but after that she faithfully made her weekly deposits at the ATM, no matter how busy her schedule became.

Preparing Monthly Financial Reports

By keeping current records of business finances, you can avoid paying too much or too little on your quarterly taxes. You'll also prevent feeling overwhelmed at the end of the year trying to piece together information for tax returns. If you use a computer financial program like Quicken and an accountant's services, your monthly financial tasks can be simple and fast (see Appendix F).

As a general practice, pay business expenses as often as possible through your business account (e.g., checks, credit card, and automatic debits). Then, when generating financial reports with business account information, important tax-deductible expenses will automatically be included. Payments will also show on credit card and bank statements, useful for future reference and if you are ever audited. Automatic debits are an efficient way to make recurring payments, saving you the time, effort, and expense of writing the same checks again and again.

Recording Cash Payments and Mileage

The few times you do pay cash for business expenses (e.g., supplies, parking fees, meals/entertainment), keep a record so you can also claim these payments as deductions. Even small expenditures quickly add up over the weeks and months, and, when claimed, will help preserve your net income. To routinely record payments, enter them in a separate area of the planner/scheduler you use for business. Manual planners usually have expense and auto mileage sheets in the back, allowing categorized entries for every day of the month. For each entry record the date, amount paid, and the expense category. To record business automobile mileage, also enter daily miles driven and destinations. Total and print or tear out these records monthly and keep them in the same folder with the bank and other financial statements.

My friend, Laura, keeps her auto mileage record and pen in her car and writes down business miles before getting out of the car at her destinations. She finds that with this method she can accurately report miles by looking at the odometer, and she doesn't have to remember to record miles later, when attending to other priorities.

Filing Log Reports

Whether you use a software program or manual system for your billing and practice management tasks, you will also have log reports which provide a weekly accounting of all the services you've provided and payments you've received for each client (see pp. 127–129). File these reports in a separate log report folder.

Sending Reports Quarterly

Once you've prepared weekly and monthly financial reports, all you need to do each quarter is access your folders and send these reports (i.e., bank, reconciliation, transaction or journals, cash/mileage, and log reports) to your accountant. In return he or she will send you financial statements and updated estimates of quarterly tax payments.

To help develop your own routine, you may wish to refer to the financial tasks checklist in Appendix F, which lists the steps we've covered to prepare deposits and financial reports.

Issue	Recommendation
Managing your practice finances.	1) To independently manage business finances, use a separate checking account, ATM and credit card, and deposit stamp for your practice (pp. 151–152).
	2) For fast access to information and automated financial reports, keep your checking account on a computer software program (e.g., Quicken) (pp. 152–153).
	3) For the most savings, order checks by mail; to maintain a healthy account balance and avoid service charges, deposit receipts weekly (pp. 153–155).
	4) To pay quarterly taxes accurately and avoid end-of-year work overload, reconcile your account and organize financial reports monthly; send reports quarterly to an accountant for updated financial statements and tax estimates (pp. 155–156).

Collecting Client Fees

By collecting client payments at the time of service, you will greatly reduce outstanding fees. However, your receipts can still be less than expected at times. In addition to overdue insurance payments, some clients will accrue fees for canceling late or not showing up for appointments. Chapter 8 helps you set up a cancellation/no-show policy and fully inform clients before they engage services, a helpful deterrent to violations and accompanying fees. However, you'll still encounter some clients who do not follow the policy; in these situations, it can be difficult and unpleasant to collect client payments. You may even prefer to ignore this aversive task. But consider that you're passing up the chance to reinforce clients' responsibility and ability to follow through and directly address relevant therapeutic issues. You'll also lose unclaimed income while feeling the stress of uncompensated services. The following steps will help you collect client payments to maximally benefit your clients and your practice.

Collect at the Beginning of Sessions

Your first step in collecting client fees is to do so at the time of service. This will save you the work and expense of mailing bills and prevent delays and uncertainties in being compensated. To allow time to deal with problems if they occur, collect fees at the beginning instead of the end of the session. Clients can sometimes forget to bring payments or take a long time to find them in their purse, wallet, or pockets. By addressing fees in the beginning, you'll have time to get compensated, solve problems, and still end sessions on time. You'll be able to fully focus on providing service and avoid the stressful distraction of anticipating last-minute payment problems. Your subsequent clients will benefit as well when their sessions start on time and you can focus on their needs without the residual stress of prior session delays.

To establish a precedent, introduce your policy in the first session after you've greeted new clients, collected forms, guided them to the therapy room, and briefly reviewed their reason for coming. You can say, "The first thing I always do in sessions is take care of fees to get them out of the way. That way we can spend the whole time talking about your concerns. As we discussed before, your payment is _____ dollars, cash or check (or credit card) will work fine." Continue to collect fees at the beginning of every subsequent session. By being consistent, clients will become familiar with this routine and may even organize payment in advance, reducing the time you'll need for this task.

I discovered the value of this payment policy after many years of collecting payments at the end of sessions. Slowly but surely my stress accumulated as intermittent problems arose just when session time ran out. Although the situations were varied and sporadic, they were cumulatively draining as sessions ended late, creating a domino effect of schedule disruption throughout the day. Sometimes people realized their checkbook was missing, others had forgotten to go to the ATM. A few had just changed purses, had just written their last check, and other unique dilemmas.

I vividly remember when I realized something had to change. I was treating a newly separated client in her late 50s named Doris, who was suffering from major depression and generalized anxiety. She was overwhelmed with being single again after thirty years of marriage, enraged with her husband for leaving her for another woman, and facing the prospect of returning to work for the first time since her 20s. Due to limited finances, Doris had just moved into a small apartment with her elderly mother, who reminded her of her critical and controlling soon-to-be ex-husband. Every time she wrote out her check at the session's end, she would pause many times, bubbling over with new issues, memories, and feelings with each pen stroke. With concern for her fragile status, I tried different calming ways to help her complete her task, but to no avail. Invariably, sessions ended late and the stress carried over to the next session, which, in turn, started late. Later that night after all sessions were finished, thankfully my inner light bulb flashed on. I realized these costs were too much; it was time to move payment to the session's beginning for everyone's sake.

The next day I started right in, telling all of my clients when they first arrived, "Instead of paying at the end of our sessions, I'd like to do it first thing to get it out of the way. That way we can spend the whole time talking about your concerns." To my surprise no one became upset with this change, and what I thought might appear a presumptuous request was taken in stride. Although Doris still paused when writing her check, this was no longer stressful as she had plenty of time to complete this task and I had plenty of time to address her concerns. Now, when other clients forget payment—and they still do—or are slow in paying, we have time in the beginning to figure out a solution. No overtime drain anymore. Those frustrating attempts to hurry people along at the last minute are gone. I can stay focused on clients' issues, no longer wasting time and energy anticipating and confronting last-minute problems.

If Clients Forget Session Payments

By stating exact fees and collecting at the beginning of sessions, you will greatly reduce the chances of clients forgetting to bring payments. However, if they do, to ensure rapid reimbursement, review the policy at the session's start and offer options to bring payment back right after the session ends or send it that day in the mail. To facilitate follow-through, provide a self-addressed envelope; if clients choose the former option, show them where they can drop payment off at your office. Both choices require clients to step out of their routine, and may help them remember to bring payments to subsequent sessions to avoid similar efforts in the future. Before their next appointment, verify that you've received payment and thank clients at the session's start for taking care of this task.

With these directives, you'll probably find that most clients take care of payment by the following session. In the rare event that they don't, address it right away and when possible, collect during that session. If necessary, repeat your directive to bring the remaining payment after the session or send it in the mail. Depending on your theoretical orientation and therapy approach, you may also wish to explore underlying issues related to clients' payment delays, incorporating them into current therapeutic work.

If Clients Drop Out with Unpaid Bills

When following collection recommendations, the only other way clients will accrue outstanding fees is by not honoring your cancellation/no-show policy. Chapter 8 describes how to address violations right away through phone calls and, when necessary, mailing initial bills. You'll probably find that the majority of continuing clients quickly take care of bills, while those who stop services are less likely to pay.

For clients who drop out and have not paid missed session fees after the first bill, you could send another written bill after a month. However, I don't generally recommend this, as your likelihood of receiving payment is small and not worth the time and effort you'd spend preparing second bills.

When first in practice I didn't know that multiple billings were a lot of work for little return. I routinely billed clients for outstanding fees up to three months in a row. I even bought flashy reminder stickers from the office supply store to place on bills to catch clients' attention. They read as follows: (Bill #2) "*YOUR ACCOUNT IS PAST DUE*. We would appreciate your payment today!"; (Bill #3) "*FINAL NOTICE*. This is the last statement that will be sent to you. Unless paid at once the account will be turned over for collection."

In time, I realized that second and third billings did not noticeably increase payments compared to billing one time. I suspect the stickers may have even turned off some people. Although the final notice sticker alluded to collection agencies, fortunately I never used their services for the reasons just described. Over time, by developing and implementing the cancellation/no-show policy detailed in Chapter 8, violations occurred less and less frequently. Now when clients incur outstanding fees and do not continue in treatment, I save time and effort by billing just once.

For the same reasons, I don't recommend using a collection agency or taking clients to small claims court. You increase the risk of clients responding by filing complaints or taking legal actions. Even if you appropriately inform clients at the outset of services about engaging these outside resources if necessary, they could later become upset when contacted about bills and pursue retaliatory actions that could make your life miserable. Consider that by consistently adhering to your payment policies, you will keep outstanding fees to a minimum. Even if you did hire an agency to collect such small amounts, after subtracting collection fees, you would have very little to show for all your effort and potential risk.

My colleague, Jack, who's been in practice over thirty years, shared that the one time he was the subject of a formal complaint was after using a collection agency to recover an unpaid client bill. He had followed all the appropriate steps to collect overdue fees, including informing his client at the outset of treatment that he used collection agencies when necessary. After making numerous attempts to collect through phone calls and mailed bills with no response, Jack engaged the collection service to recover fees.

Soon after, he was informed by his state licensing board that there was a complaint filed against him by the client, alleging he violated confidentiality in using the collection agency. Jack had all the evidence to support his actions, copies of the informed consent signed by the client, the bills he had mailed, logged attempts to call the client, and detailed records of services and unpaid fees. The complaint was dismissed, but only after a stressful process that lasted over a year. Jack spent numerous hours responding to investigation inquiries, preparing written statements, and appearing at the licensing hearing. Although he prevailed, the initial complaint remained on record, so whenever he applied to join a professional organization or insurance company panel, he had to document the complaint on every application.

In sum, it's been my experience that it has not been worth the costs required to pursue unpaid bills for clients who have discontinued services.

Recording Outstanding Fees

By routinely recording missed visits, charges, and payments, you can easily review clients' payment history if they reinitiate services in the future. The longer you practice in one location, the more likely you are to encounter clients who return for services. By checking for outstanding bills before returning inquiry calls, you can address them before clients resume sessions, reinforcing their responsibility to follow through with payment. This may be therapeutic for clients who are habitually unreliable in other areas of their lives. You'll also reclaim lost income, even if it's been a year or longer after you last saw the client. Plus, by immediately attending to bills, you can help to prevent a pattern of repeat violations.

Method

To record missed sessions, use the same computer or manual system you normally use to log and bill client sessions. Add a separate entry for each client's missed visit including the date, name, service, fee, adjustment, amount charged, and payment. The service will either be a client no-show (e.g., NS) or late cancellation (e.g., C). For quick reference later, add whether this is a first or later missed session, the client's reason, and basis for fee adjustments. A typical ledger entry might look something like this:

Date	Name	Service	Fee	Adj.	Charge	Payment
12/5/04	Johnson, Rachel	C	$100	$20	$80	$0

Notes: C#1, states forgot appt, charged contracted insurance rate.

Upon receiving payments for missed visit fees, record these also in individual ledger entries. Most software programs offer the option to automatically calculate and add interest to overdue fees. However, I wouldn't recommend this, as it can be offensive to clients and more work than it's worth. You would have to notify clients before beginning the practice of charging interest, and deal with negative reactions if they become upset after receiving bills with interest charges. When you adhere to payment policies, outstanding fees will be small and interest will be insignificant. Rather than charging interest, your clients and your practice will be better served by spending your time and energy on other activities with more potential for reward.

Issue	Recommendation
Collecting client fees.	1) To efficiently solve payment problems as well as to stay focused on service and keep appointments on time, collect client fees at the beginning (versus the end) of sessions (pp. 157–159). 2) To facilitate follow-through if clients forget payments, direct them to drop off your fee after the session ends or send it that day in the mail (pp. 159–160). 3) To prevent spending time and effort for little return, send only one bill to clients who've stopped services, and do not engage outside collection agencies or small claims courts (pp. 160–161). 4) To address outstanding fees if clients reinitiate services later, routinely record missed sessions; to avoid offending clients and fruitless work, do not charge interest for overdue bills (pp. 161–162).

If Clients Return with Unpaid Bills

If you discover overdue fees for returning clients, address this over the phone before setting a new appointment. In general, do not immediately offer payment breaks, since clients have already broken policy through no-shows and lack of payment. Direct clients instead to pay the full amount (e.g., "You do have an outstanding fee of ninety dollars from missing your last scheduled appointment. You can either pay this now by mailing cash or a check, or you can bring it to our appointment. Which would you like to do?"). If you are concerned that certain fragile clients may be affected negatively, wait and discuss this in person in the first return session.

After hearing about past-due fees, some clients may decide not to pursue services. Depending on your preference, you may wish to thera-peutically address their reactions. Other clients may request extra time or price breaks in paying off overdue bills. For people in financial distress for which full payment would present a hardship, you could give them a break and offer a payment plan (see pp. 191–192). This allows clients more time to pay old bills while holding them responsible for the total charge. If you offer this break, do so only for previous outstanding bills. This will preserve and reinforce your policy that payments are due in full at the beginning of each session.

If Clients Return and Repeat Violations

You'll probably find that most returning clients do not have unpaid bills. However, some may incur new cancellation fees and upon review you might discover that they did the same thing in previous treatment. As with any policy violation, address it right away to help prevent future breaches. The simplest approach is to charge the full fee for the missed visit (see pp. 175–176).

If you want to offer payment breaks, make sure one year has passed between the previous violation to the current one before offering a break. By following this timeframe you will ensure that clients who break policy more than once in a year are fully accountable for missed session fees. This guideline also reinforces the value of your services, helping to preserve your professional self-esteem and positive regard for clients. If you prefer, you can modify the timeframe to suite your preferences and individual client situations.

My colleague, David, provided services for a teenage boy named Adam and his parents. Adam had stopped hanging out with his friends, was skip-ping basketball practice, his grades had dropped, and he was staying in his room and sleeping excessively. Whenever his parents tried to talk with him, he became angry and told them he didn't want to talk about anything. He reluctantly agreed to attend therapy and was supposed to drive on his own to meet his parents at David's office, but he did not show for the first session. After using the session to share their concerns with David, Adam's parents talked with him again and he agreed to attend therapy. This time they drove him to the session and fortunately he bonded well with David. After ruling out substance abuse, David assessed that Adam had become depressed after a breakup with a girlfriend. He helped Adam process this loss individually and then briefly with his parents, which helped Adam regain his confidence and self-esteem. After a few individual and family sessions, Adam was back to his old self and had already met a new girl he liked.

A few years later, Adam sought services from David on his own, remembering how helpful therapy had been. He was finishing his last year of college, and was stressed and confused about his future. He had just broken up with his girlfriend, and although he had initiated the break, he was still upset about the loss. Before calling Adam back, David checked his history and noted that Adam had missed a session in past therapy. During the return call David followed normal protocol in reviewing his cancellation policy and fee with Adam.

Adam attended the first session, but he did not show for the second. Although the missed visit was years after the prior violation, David decided not to offer a break and charged his full missed session fee. Adam called back and apologized, explaining that he had forgotten the appointment. He paid the fee and continued with services until he felt better about ending his relationship and had sorted through options to plan for his future. He did not miss an appointment again. By enforcing policy right away, David helped to prevent a pattern of no-shows and facilitated Adam's follow-through in getting the help he needed.

Factors to Consider when Collecting Fees

There are many factors to consider when enforcing your policies and collecting fees. They include client factors, your reactions, and additional factors specific to your practice.

Client Factors

Clients who incur outstanding fees may have done this in prior therapy somewhere else with no consequences (e.g., an agency with no policies or lax collections). Some clients may assume that you operate like other professionals they see who do not charge fees for policy violations. For example, many busy physician's offices book clients every fifteen minutes and do not enforce a cancellation policy, as there is always an overflow of people waiting for sessions.

Other clients may violate policy because they are overwhelmed with the stressors and/or clinical symptoms that bring them into therapy. And some clients may have difficulty maintaining structure and follow-through in many areas of their lives. Personality features can also contribute to violations (e.g., issues with authority, testing of boundaries).

Cancellation and collection policies will help you therapeutically deal with these and other client factors. They reinforce client consistency, responsibility, and accountability, and serve as a useful extension of the therapy you are already providing. By calmly adhering to the rules, you also model stability and predictability. Clients are encouraged to take responsibility by paying fees they incur and to honor commitments in the future by following policy guidelines. For many people the message reinforced is to keep their needs and scheduled appointments a priority, even when others place last-minute demands on their time and attention.

My colleague, Tom, quickly realized the value of enforcing his cancellation policy when his client, Sandra, called at the last minute to cancel her session. Sandra had suffered from severe depression all her life and was referred to Tom for psychotherapy by her prescribing psychiatrist. Her symptoms had worsened in the last two years as she became overwhelmed with multiple demands from her full-time job, children, husband, and extended family. It was hard for her to say no to anyone, so she spent almost all of her time attending to everyone's needs but her own. Her husband and children had become accustomed to her attention and expected her to drop everything when they requested.

The day she cancelled her session, her husband had asked her at the last minute to stay home with him and the children, and as usual, she had quickly agreed. Soon after she called to cancel, Tom called Sandra back, reminding her of the cancellation policy and fee. Sandra shared this with her husband and he quickly changed his mind about wanting her to stay home, as he did not relish the idea of paying the full fee for Sandra's missed appointment.

When Sandra arrived at her session, Tom therapeutically addressed her decision to cancel, relating it to a general pattern of forgoing her own needs at her expense. By enforcing the cancellation policy, he helped

Sandra see that she deserved to set boundaries to preserve her time and attend to her needs. Although Tom had to enforce policy a few more times, each time Sandra was able to reprioritize her needs and keep her appointment. She also started setting more boundaries on the job and with her children, and even joined a women's gym. As of the last update, she was exercising three times a week and had lost thirty pounds. She had also just completed laser eye surgery, something she had always wanted but until then did not feel she deserved.

Sometimes violations will reflect clients' resistance to current therapeutic work. Enforcing policy can facilitate a turning point, helping clients decide whether to fully engage in therapy or to stop services. If someone does drop out, you can offer that time to another client more likely to benefit from your services. You'll avoid the problem of people who show up half the time, do not work consistently in therapy, and leave you with holes of uncompensated time in your schedule.

I had been working with my client, Margaret, for a few weeks when she began a pattern of calling at the last minute to cancel. She initially came to therapy requesting stress-management skills to help cope with her demanding job as a nurse care manager. She responded well and was soon able to lower her stress on the job. In the course of treatment, she shared that she had been physically abused as a child by her parents, and had never addressed or emotionally healed from this trauma. She decided that this was a good time to finally confront old wounds even though it would be hard.

An hour or so before her next two sessions, she called to cancel. Each time I called her right back and reminded her of the cancellation policy, and both times she managed to adjust her schedule to attend the sessions. We talked about her ambivalence in confronting her painful past and each time she decided to continue this therapy focus. The next week she cancelled at the last minute again and was not available when I returned her call. Because she did not make it to the appointment, I followed policy and charged her the missed session fee.

This was Margaret's turning point; she scheduled another session and paid the outstanding fee. We continued to focus on healing her trauma and with the help of policy enforcements, she stayed committed and consistent in therapy. She fully processed her trauma; no longer was it a scary monster lurking in the back of her mind. Her attempts to forget what happened evolved into anger, sadness, and eventually love for the brave, resourceful little girl who had not only survived but also thrived.

Your Reactions

When clients break policies, your reactions could also compromise your services and enforcements. One danger of waiving your policies is that you can start feeling negatively toward your clients. Over time your stress from disrupted treatment and uncompensated time can spill over to interactions with clients and decrease the effectiveness of your clinical work. By following policies, you'll help to prevent this stress from building and preserve the quality of your services.

If you are new to practice and building a client base you may be afraid of alienating clients and losing them with restrictive rules. You may assume that by flexing your policies, clients will be more likely to continue in therapy. For example, you might repeatedly allow people to miss visits with no fee. However, consider that clients may still drop out of therapy whether breaks are given or not. And it's possible that the more flexible you are with ongoing clients, the more likely they will repeat policy breaches.

When I was getting started in practice, I was afraid that clients would become upset and stop coming if I appeared too rigid in enforcing policies. I assumed that flexing policies would preserve rapport and enhance therapeutic effectiveness. I often let clients slide when they called at the last minute to cancel or did not show for appointments. To my surprise, what I thought was the best approach lead to the opposite of what I expected. The very clients to whom I had offered breaks frequently repeated policy violations and I felt more stressed each time. I started to have negative feelings about these clients during sessions, and soon became aware that treatment could suffer as a result.

After realizing things were getting worse with my lenient approach, I faced my fears of clients' reactions and enforced policies. It was uncomfortable at first, and some clients that I had previously been flexible with became upset. However, with time I became more comfortable enforcing policies, and clients responded in kind. My negative reactions to clients disappeared and my professional self-worth and confidence grew. With fewer disruptions, therapy became more productive and my income and time were preserved. Now most people honor policies, and those who don't quickly learn through enforcement and are less likely to do it again. The rare client who drops out frees time for someone else to be seen.

Other Factors

Another factor to consider when enforcing policies is your client population. For example, if many of your clients are chronically ill, they may cancel at the last minute or not show more often than healthy clients because of a rapid decline in their condition that day. You may decide to flex policy more often or respond the same to these clients as your healthier ones. Whatever you do, be sure you are comfortable with your decision; you will prevent feeling negatively toward your clients and maintain the effectiveness of your services.

My colleague, Brian, works with many clients who are chronically ill and covered through the same worker's compensation insurance carrier. Some days his clients wake up so physically sick that they cannot even get out of bed. When clients cancel sessions at the last minute due to their deteriorated physical condition, Brian offers shorter phone consultations instead. Before providing this option, he checked whether the insurance plan would cover this service. He knew that many traditional carriers did not pay for phone visits, but he thought the worker's compensation insurance might be different. He learned that as long as he provided additional documentation, the carrier did cover this service, if billed through specific phone consultation codes. His chronically ill clients now receive the treatment they need regardless of their physical condition and Brian is reimbursed for all the services he provides.

Even when you set policies, unexpected situations can still pop up that derail your enforcements. Just when you think you have devised a system that ensures compliance while preserving ongoing therapy, someone may react completely differently (e.g., dropping out of therapy, skipping payment). When you have done your best to enforce policy and a client still has not come through, be as kind to yourself as you can. Tell yourself, "It's okay, I did what I could and this person just did not respond." Instead of expecting 100 percent compliance, you can hope that a majority of clients will honor your policies, the rest you can release.

Some clients still surprise me in my practice and I suspect this will happen at times no matter what I do. For example, I granted my client, Lisa, a first-time break by offering a payment plan for her cancellation fee. She agreed to pay an extra ten dollars each session until her outstanding fee was paid. After the second payment Lisa called well in advance to cancel her next appointment, saying she would call back to reschedule once her finances were in better shape. A few days later her last check was returned for insufficient funds along with an extra bank charge of four dollars. I sent Lisa a bill right away for the outstanding fees and included a copy of the bank statement for the bounced check. Although I could have billed again, I decided the work and time I'd spend were not worth the small chance of getting paid. I did not receive any more payments or contacts for future appointments and to this day she has an outstanding fee. Although the situation was frustrating at the time, I reminded myself that I did what I could and Lisa just didn't respond. However, if she does call for another appointment, before calling back I will review her treatment and payment history. I'll quickly find her overdue fee and address it with her before she reschedules another session.

Issue	Recommendation
Factors to consider when enforcing policies and collecting fees.	1) To prevent repeat policy violations, address outstanding fees with returning clients and new bills with current clients right away (pp. 163–164). 2) To therapeutically enhance clients' responsibility, self-care, and release of treatment resistance, consistently enforce cancellation and collection policies (pp. 164–166). 3) To preserve treatment effectiveness, enforce policies even if you fear clients' negative reactions and attrition (p. 167). 4) To preserve quality service if you flex policy, be sure you are comfortable with your decision; to reduce stress when clients do not respond to policy enforcements, forgo additional efforts to pursue outstanding fees (pp. 167–169).

CHAPTER EIGHT

Implementing a Successful Cancellation Policy

Last-minute cancellations and no-shows are a major hazard in private practice. With each missed session, treatment is disrupted, rescheduling takes time and effort, and practice income is lost. Imagine that you've just finished preparing a timely intervention for your client. At the last minute she calls to leave a message that she can't come to her session because her boyfriend surprised her with a visit. Or, picture yourself sitting in your office waiting for a couple that doesn't show or call to explain what happened. If you've already experienced a similar scenario, you know what a burden these situations can be.

One of the best ways to prevent these stressors is to develop and implement a cancellation policy in your practice. This chapter helps you to create a policy and introduce it to clients before therapy starts. You will learn how to provide multiple reminders to help clients follow the protocol. You will also receive a range of options to enforce your policy. By following these steps, you will proactively reduce last-minute cancellations and no-shows and efficiently deal with them if they do occur.

Certainly real emergencies can and do happen to cause missed sessions. One such crisis happened to my client, Rebecca, a single mother of three. She was rushed to the emergency room the morning of her scheduled appointment when her autoimmune disorder (Sweet's Syndrome) took a life-threatening turn for the worse. Fortunately, Rebecca made it to the hospital in time for critical treatment and was able to go home a few days later. In a situation like this, there is no question of an emergency.

However, what you are more likely to encounter are people who give a variety of non-urgent reasons for missing their sessions. Some typical examples include an executive whose business meeting runs late, a student who decides to attend a study group, a parent who can't find child care, a couple who mix up their schedules, and many more.

Consider, too, that in self-employed private practice your income is directly linked to how many clients you see that day. This is very different from traditional employment in clinics or institutions in which you are paid a salary regardless of how much direct care you provide. As a private practitioner, insurance companies do not pay for unattended appointments and you have no guaranteed backup to reclaim losses.

When I started in private practice, I became acutely aware of the shift from steady to variable reimbursements. Before becoming self-employed, I reacted very calmly when clients missed visits at my salaried Veterans Administration job. I even welcomed the extra time, using it to write reports, return phone calls, and consult with colleagues. However, once I started working for myself, I became intensely aware of losing income with every missed session.

Next to dealing with insurance, late cancellations and no-shows were the most stressful aspect to private practice, particularly when people offered casual reasons for missing. At first I waived policy and cancellation fees but I noticed that the more I gave clients a break, the more violations occurred. Through these tribulations I tried different approaches to stop this pattern, and over the years those that worked have become the most valuable strategies I use in everyday practice. I believe they can do the same for you, preserving your treatment, saving you time and grief, and protecting your bottom line.

A Sample Policy

To help clients understand and remember your cancellation policy, keep it as simple and clear as possible. One standard policy you can use requires clients to cancel at least twenty-four hours before their scheduled session or they will be charged the entire fee for the missed visit. A one-day cancellation timeframe has the advantage of appearing reasonable and not too difficult for people to follow. If you prefer, you could substitute forty-eight or seventy-two hours, or a different option individualized to your practice.

Using Multiple Reminders

To enhance compliance from the beginning, explain your policy to clients over the phone when you are arranging for the first appointment (see Chapter 4). To formalize the agreement, include the policy in the treatment consent form you give clients to read and sign in the first session (see Appendix D). By placing the policy on the page that clients sign and date, they are more likely to read it when completing the form. The policy could read as follows:

Canceled/Missed Appointments
A scheduled appointment means that time is reserved only for you. If an appointment is missed or canceled with less than twenty-four–hours notice, you will be billed directly according to the scheduled fee or according to the rules of your health plan. Your health plan does not cover payment for missed appointments; therefore, you are responsible for payment in full.

Reminding High-Risk Clients

If you suspect that any clients are at risk for breaking the policy, add a verbal reminder in the first session or as soon as you can. Pull out the consent form and direct clients to look at the policy and read it to them. You might ask, "Do you have any questions about the consent form you signed? One part I'd like to reinforce is the cancellation policy right here (read the policy out loud). Do you have any questions about that?"

Your clinical judgment can help you identify warning signs of potential violators, such as clients with simultaneous work or school absences, recurring crises, severe clinical symptoms, certain personality features, etc. The most common red flags I find are borderline and histrionic personality features. When one of my new clients, an art instructor, brought a bag of limes to her first session for payment, I knew right away there could be trouble. Years ago my friend and fellow intern showed me a huge bag of homemade bagels her chronic pain client and baker had dropped off as payment to her. It was so big she could barely lift it. Although some clues may not be as obvious as these, by staying alert you can begin to sense warning signals common to your practice to help you reinforce policy again and again.

For clients you are very concerned about, give them a copy of the consent form to take-home as another tangible reminder. The first appointment can be frightening and overwhelming for many people; they are often completely focused on their concerns and don't even process procedural details. Others may be so compromised by their presenting symptoms that they are barely functioning at all (e.g., those with bipolar disorder, severe depression, or posttraumatic stress disorder, to name a few).

My office neighbor, Melanie, discovered one of her new clients suffering a severe panic attack in the waiting room; the client could not sign the consent form because her hands were shaking so much. Another was so depressed, he did not turn the first page over to complete the second and third signature page underneath. By checking their forms, Melanie helped them read and sign the entire document, including the cancellation policy, and made a copy for them to take-home. With clients like these, multiple reminders can be crucial to helping them understand and honor your cancellation policy.

Appointment Cards

Another way to reinforce policy is through future appointment cards. They are inexpensive, small and convenient, and can be purchased at most office supply sources. Clients can put them in their wallet, purse, car, on their refrigerator, and other places as reminders. Most card styles offer the option to include a statement of your cancellation policy at the bottom, for example:

> If unable to keep appointment kindly give twenty-four–hours notice.

At the end of each session, give clients an appointment card and direct them to fill in the day and time of their next appointment. When people make written, public commitments they are more likely to follow through. By watching clients as they complete the cards, you will help them attend the sessions they commit to and honor the cancellation policy if they cannot. To avoid miscommunications, make sure they fill in the correct date and time.

Many clients have told me they refer to their appointment cards often, and some have narrowly avoided no-shows after finding a card in their purse or wallet. One harried mother told me she was at the store and opened her checkbook to discover her appointment card with her scheduled time the next hour. She was able to get her errand done and rush over, avoiding a costly no-show. Another busy executive always transferred his appointment information to his electronic organizer, keeping the card in his wallet as a backup reminder.

Appointment cards may also provide a tangible extension of therapeutic support and progress. They can remind clients of therapy goals, insights, progress, and steps they need to take. Additionally, whenever people glance at the cards, another reminder of the cancellation policy is there for them to read.

I once worked with a saleswoman who wanted help with a public speaking phobia. She was preparing for an upcoming sales talk and was very anxious about presenting in front of a group. Part of her therapy included a self-calming exercise. One step was to identify a cue word she could use to engage her favorite relaxing memory of walking on the beach in the morning. She chose *tranquil* and wrote it down as a reminder on every appointment card. Whenever she looked at it, she reinforced her relaxation response. Plus, the cancellation policy was right below.

During her therapy she honored the cancellation policy, calling in advance to reschedule appointments when they conflicted with out-of-town sales trips. More importantly, when she gave her sales talk, she was able to remain calm the entire time. By attending sessions consistently, she had become so good at self-calming that she imagined the entire audience in their underwear, much to her delight.

Even when cards are lost, they can still help clients honor your policy. Clients may call when they can't find their card to ask when their appointment is scheduled. If they call before their scheduled session, they can usually make it on time. Even if clients call too late to attend, they are more likely to honor the cancellation policy fee when they've previously committed to appointments by filling out the cards.

Your cancellation policy and reminders can also help in ways you don't even expect at just the right time. Clients are more likely to call ahead to cancel, freeing sessions for others in need of being seen.

One day my former client, Alison, left a brief and pleasant message requesting an appointment. In prior treatment she had requested services for grieving and life transition issues. She was struggling after her mother's sudden death, a recent relocation to a new state with her boyfriend, and being unemployed after ten years of full-time work. By the end of therapy Alison had become engaged and was planning her wedding, she was working in a new full-time job, and her grief for her mother was not so overwhelming.

After checking messages between sessions, I jotted her number down and looked at my schedule—nothing available for two weeks. I proceeded with the next appointment and afterward checked again for new calls. Someone scheduled for 1 P.M. the next day had just called to cancel, requesting to come the following week instead. I called Alison right away and offered her the open time.

Although she did not reveal any distress over the phone, Alison was in a major crisis, having just found out after returning from her honeymoon that her new husband had been lying to her and abusing cocaine for over a year. Through immediate intervention, she was able to confront him with her intention to leave if he did not get help. He agreed and entered a substance abuse program, where he continues to receive follow-up treatment. Although many situations may not be as dramatic as this, setting and reinforcing a cancellation policy can produce big benefits just when they are needed.

Issue	Recommended Approaches
Increasing compliance with your cancellation policy.	1) To enhance compliance from the beginning, introduce and review your policy during the client's inquiry call (pp. 170–172, 95–96). 2) To formalize the agreement, include your cancellation policy in the treatment consent form that the client reads and signs (p. 172). 3) To remind clients at high risk for violations, read the cancellation policy out loud and give the client a copy to take home (pp. 172–173). 4) To provide a tangible policy reminder and facilitate treatment, direct the client to fill out a future appointment card to take home (pp. 173–175).

Enforcement

Sometimes after following all the recommended steps to introduce and reinforce your policy, people will still not show or cancel at the last minute. The simplest way to respond is to directly follow the policy and charge the full fee for a missed session. Before charging insured clients, make sure your contract with the insurance carrier does not prohibit billing clients for missed visits. If you don't have quick access to your contract, call the insurance company and speak with an agent in the provider relations or billing department to verify the no-show billing policy.

Almost all carriers allow billing clients for missed visits. In fact, most clearly state that clients are responsible for paying for no-shows. However, once in awhile you'll find an insurance plan that does not. For example, some employee assistance provider (EAP) contracts through managed care companies do not allow you to bill clients for no-shows.

Charge Your Contracted Rates

For insured clients, match cancellation fees with your contracted rate with their company, usually lower than your normal session fee. For example, if your normal session fee is $100 and your contracted rate is eighty dollars, charge the client eighty dollars for a missed session. Ethically, you'll avoid taking advantage of clients because you won't receive more than insurance would pay if they had attended the session. Legally, many insurance provider contracts require that you continue billing clients your contracted rates if you continue treatment beyond benefit limits. By charging contracted rates for missed visit fees, clients' bills will always comply with fee schedules if there are ever any questions or complaints from clients or anyone else.

Address Policy Violations

If you don't hear from clients who've missed sessions, call as soon as possible to remind them of the cancellation policy and fee they incurred. Sometimes people will call right away to explain their no-show. Imagine that your client, Sally, did not show for her weekly appointment and called soon after to say she completely forgot. You can say, "Since there is a twenty-four–hour cancellation policy (and insurance doesn't pay for missed visits), your fee will be eighty dollars. I know you are very responsible and will take care of this. You can send the fee for the missed session in the mail now, drop it off at the office, or bring it to the next visit. Which would you like to do?"

Here you give Sally a choice in how to handle payment and whether to schedule another session. You also affirm your trust in her. When you show faith in clients' responsibility and trustworthiness, they are more likely to see themselves that way too and act accordingly—in this situation, by paying their bill.

Your Delivery

When reviewing and enforcing your cancellation policy, approach the discussions in as unbiased a tone as possible. When your delivery is matter-of-fact versus angry or displeased, you'll help avoid destructive reactions. Some clients who violate rules may be unconsciously testing you for a negative emotional response. When you treat every interaction with clients as an extension of therapy, it will be easier to stay in a neutral role, especially when dealing with uncomfortable policy and payment issues. You'll preserve therapeutic rapport and structure and feel less stressed, both emotionally and physically.

When Clients Do Not Reschedule

For clients who do not schedule a future appointment, confirm whether they will mail the payment or drop it off at the office. Provide specific directions to help them follow through and to ensure the payment does not get lost. If clients choose to mail the payment, make sure they write down your correct address. If they plan to drop off the fee at your office, tell them what to do. Imagine that your client, Sally, further explains her no-show. She tells you that she has become so busy with her part-time job and three children's activities that something has to give and unfortunately it is her therapy. With your help she is feeling much better now and she would like to see how things go on her own. She thanks you for all your help and plans to drop the payment off at your office. After expressing support and understanding you could say, "Please put the payment in an envelope, seal it, write my name on the outside, and then slide it under my office door. So I'll know when to look for it, when do you plan to come by?"

If Clients Request Bills

Some clients may ask for a bill detailing the missed session and fee before making their payment. If so, send a computer-generated, typed, or written statement as soon as possible. Do this also for clients whom you cannot reach by phone. If you use a computer billing program (see Chapter 6), you can easily create and print these bills. If not, generate your own bills including the client's name and address, the date of service, the fee charged and brief explanation, and your name and address.

My colleague, Susan, uses personalized "double duty" statement/envelopes for her client bills. Her name and address are printed on the envelope and inside there is a blank section to fill in billing details. When people open the envelope they can read the statement and then detach it and use the remaining self-addressed remittance envelope to pay the bill. You can find these statement/envelopes in most office supply stores.

Add Handwritten Notes

Before sending bills to clients, add a handwritten note. Clients will appreciate your personal effort, and those who've stopped services may feel more comfortable returning in the future. Include a review of payment responsibilities, your trust that clients will take care of the fee, and a direct invitation for future contact. For future reference, copy the bill and place it in the client's file. A typical note could read as follows:

> Dear Bill,
> I hope you are doing well and wish you the best in your future. I've enjoyed working with you and helping you take steps toward your goals. Thanks for sending payment of eighty dollars for the missed session to me at the above address at your earliest convenience. I know you are very responsible and will take care of this in the best way. If you have any questions feel free to call and, as always, I remain available if you would like another appointment.
> Sincerely,
> Helen Lee, MFT

After I started including personal notes with bills, I noticed that clients were more likely to respond. In addition to sending payments, some people wrote about new events in their lives and/or progress toward their goals. Clients were also more likely to return for services, sometimes months or years later.

One thing to leave off of written bills is another reminder of the cancellation policy for future visits. Clients could interpret a written policy reminder as a punitive, angry statement and react negatively. They may have experienced controlling, judging authority figures in the past and adopted a rebellious or avoidant response to similarly perceived attacks. By carefully wording bills you can prevent your notes from appearing harsh and avoid miscommunications. If clients call for another appointment, you can remind them of the cancellation policy over the phone, where you can deliver the message calmly, monitor clients' reactions, and respond therapeutically if necessary.

Issue	Recommendation
Addressing cancellation policy violations.	1) To directly follow policy, charge clients the full fee for cancellation policy violations (pp. 175–176).
	2) To prevent destructive reactions, remind clients of the policy and fee owed in a calm, non-confrontational manner (p. 177).
	3) To facilitate payment when clients do not schedule another appointment, give specific directions to mail or drop off the missed session fee (pp. 177–178).
	4) To preserve rapport and encourage follow-through in payment, add a personal, handwritten note to client bills (p. 178).

Additional Options

Sometimes you may want to bend your cancellation policy based on the client, the situation, your personal style, or any other factor. The following choices offer ways you can be flexible with your policy and still follow general guidelines. If you choose any of these options, share them only at the time you offer them to clients. This will prevent clients from expecting policy breaks and allow you the discretion to follow the policy exactly or bend it if you choose.

Grace Period

Some clients may call to cancel their appointment in advance but miss the twenty-four–hour deadline. Although technically this violates your policy, you could be flexible based on how close to the twenty-four–hour mark they call. For example, you could allow a grace period of two hours. If clients call between twenty-two and twenty-four hours in advance, allow them to cancel with no charge; if they call less than twenty-two hours ahead, enforce the policy. Consider that clients may understand the need to call the day before to cancel, but they may not always time it exactly right. A two-hour grace period allows you to bend policy for people whose calls fall just beyond the cancellation timeframe.

If you choose, you can flex the grace period even more in certain situations. For instance, my friend Laura's long-term client, a hospital technician with many personal and family stressors, called at 12:15 P.M. to cancel his session the following morning at 9 A.M. He was starting to feel ill and didn't know if he would be better by the next day.

Although the call was made after the two-hour grace period and Laura could have enforced the policy, she reviewed his individual situation and history to help decide what to do. Since he called close to the two-hour mark, had a long history of attendance, and was dealing with an emerging physical illness, Laura expanded the grace period in this situation and waived the fee. If this were my client, I would have done the same thing. Whenever you encounter gray areas like this, by using your clinical judgment and considering such factors, you can adjust your policy to best fit the individual client and situation.

Timeframe

One factor to consider when flexing your grace period (gp) is whether you have enough time after a cancellation to offer the spot to someone else. This allows those on a waiting list or new clients who call to begin services. It also preserves your income by filling an otherwise uncompensated hour. For example, it may be a very different situation if your client calls at 3 P.M. (gp = 6 hours) versus 10 P.M. (gp = 13 hours) to cancel a 9 A.M. appointment the next day. Assuming normal business hours of 9 A.M. to 5 P.M., in the former case you have two hours that day to fill the open spot while in the latter case you have no time to offer the morning appointment. One way to limit how far to flex your grace period is to allow clients to cancel up until 2 or 3 P.M. the day before an appointment. You then have two or three hours before the close of business to offer the open spot to someone else.

You can also adjust this timeframe to fit your individual practice hours. For example, if you routinely call clients in the evenings you may be comfortable occasionally flexing the grace period beyond 3 P.M., since you have more time to offer appointments to others in need. My former suitemate, Denise, routinely returns calls as late as 8 P.M., after her last session of the day. She likes making calls after 5 P.M. because she finds more people available at later times. Whatever you decide, by ensuring time to fill open hours, you are helping clients and your practice.

One-Time Exception

If you decide to flex the twenty-four–hour policy and offer a grace period, present it as a one-time exception to the policy. This lets clients know you are giving them a break and reinforces that they need to cancel twenty-four–hours in advance in the future to avoid a charge.

Imagine that your client, Joe, calls at 2 P.M. to cancel his appointment for 9 A.M. the following day, nineteen hours advance notice. After reviewing his situation, history, and other factors, you decide to allow this five-hour grace period and flex the twenty-four–hour policy this one time. You call Joe back, review the twenty-four–hour rule, and as a one-time break offer to reschedule at no charge. Before finishing, you remind him again of the policy. Here is how such a call might go:

> Hi Joe. I got your message about canceling tomorrow's appointment and just wanted to remind you of the twenty-four–hour cancellation policy. Because you called less than twenty-four hours in advance to change your session, normally I would charge the full fee. However, since this is your first time doing this and you are a very responsible person, I'd like to give you a one-time break and offer another appointment with no charge. However, if you cancel again less than twenty-four hours ahead, I will need to follow policy and charge the full fee for the missed visit.

You'll probably find that most clients are very grateful for this break, schedule another appointment, and with the added reminder are less likely to repeat this violation.

Weekends

You may also encounter people who call over the weekend to cancel their Monday appointment. If you only return calls during business hours you will have very little time to schedule someone else in an available Monday spot. In these situations, you could contact people during the weekend to fill open hours; however, after doing so you may start getting calls at any time from the very clients you've called. Assuming you don't want to return calls during personal time, you'll have to call clients back and remind them of your policy of returning routine calls during business hours. However, clients will get the message that there is a double-standard: It's okay for you to call them during weekends but it's not okay for them to call you. They may become upset, therapeutic rapport could decline, and your treatment could be affected.

This happened to me early in practice. Clients I called over the weekend to offer Monday appointments to would assume I was available to talk with them outside of business hours. When calling them back and reinforcing that I would return future calls during business hours, therapeutic rapport and treatment was sometimes affected and took time to regain. Now I make routine calls to clients only during business hours, even when Monday appointments become available.

Another strategy that helps to reduce weekend cancellations altogether, is to directly ask clients to call by Friday to cancel their Monday session. After reviewing the twenty-four–hour cancellation policy, the request could go as follows:

> Although technically you can still call twenty-four hours ahead to cancel your Monday appointment, could you please let me know by noon on Friday if you need to cancel?

Your personal preference in returning calls may differ. If you normally make calls during evenings or weekends, you may want to return client calls at these times. Whatever you choose, you can greatly reduce misunderstandings, upsets, and even dropouts by being clear and consistent about your availability.

Issue	Recommendation
Allowing a grace period for clients who cancel late but near the policy deadline.	1) To allow clients to cancel appointments near the policy deadline with no charge, allow a grace period (e.g., 2 hours), which you can adjust based on the client's situation and history (pp. 179–180). 2) To ensure enough time to offer cancelled appointments to other clients, set upper limits to your grace period based on your practice hours (p. 180). 3) To prevent repeat violations, offer the grace period to clients as a one-time policy exception (p. 181). 4) To reduce weekend cancellations and unfilled Monday sessions, directly ask Monday clients to cancel by Friday at noon (pp. 181–182).

Reminder Calls

If clients do not initially appear for appointments, you can help them make it to their session by placing a reminder call after five or ten minutes. When this works, you preserve treatment, your schedule, and save your client the cancellation fee. For example, imagine if you called your client Sally right away to remind her of her appointment when she did not show. You just might have reached her and helped her avoid the missed visit altogether.

Although this may seem like jumping the gun, with initial appointments you generally direct clients to arrive fifteen to twenty minutes before their session starts. When you call five or ten minutes into the session time it is actually twenty to twenty-five minutes after they are supposed to arrive to fill out paperwork. In subsequent sessions it's helpful to call right away so clients have time to get to your office. If people live or work nearby the odds are even better of quickly getting to a session and avoiding a no-show.

My former officemate, Karen, works with a woman, Tanya, who has struggled with severe attention deficit disorder all her life. Tanya has been so disabled by chronic lateness and forgetfulness that she has been fired from jobs, received arrest warrants for unpaid traffic tickets, filed for bankruptcy, and lost more than one boyfriend. Even with medication prescribed by her psychiatrist, she still struggles every day. Karen's reminder calls have been essential to helping Tanya attend therapy consistently and receive the treatment she so desperately needs.

If you have more than one client number (e.g., home, work, cell phone, pager) call each one to increase your chances of reaching your client. If no one answers and there is private voicemail, leave a message at each number with their scheduled appointment time and your phone number. To protect confidentiality, keep your message brief and leave out your title (e.g., psychotherapist, Dr.). For example, "This is Janet Smith, it's Wednesday at 3:05 P.M. and I have us down for a 3 o'clock appointment today. I hope everything's okay and that you're on your way. My number is _____. I look forward to seeing you soon."

Some people will be present but are screening their calls. When you leave a message you alert them right away of their visit. They can either pick up the phone and talk with you or simply come to the session even if they are late. Some clients will already be on their way when you call and show up shortly afterward; other times they may be lost finding your office and take longer to arrive.

My new client, Beth, referred with many health problems and severe depression, did not show for her first session. Luckily I found her right away by calling her cellular phone. She had confused the directions and had been driving around for quite some time looking for my office. By guiding her to the office over the phone, Beth was able to attend the rest of her session.

Fee Review

When making reminder calls, review the cancellation policy and the exact fee charged if the client misses the visit. When clients are reminded of specifically how much they will owe, they may be more motivated to make it to the session to avoid this fee: "Since there is the twenty-four–hour cancellation policy, if you don't make it to the appointment (unfortunately insurance doesn't pay for missed visits and) you will be charged the full fee of $100. You can either pay this or, since it's early in your session, you still have time to make it to the appointment and avoid this fee."

I began adding a fee review to reminder calls after clients who violated policy said they thought their fee was only their co-pay and not the entire charge. These clients had insurance and were used to paying only a portion of the session fee. Even though they were told verbally and in writing of the policy and the entire missed session fee, some still assumed their liability would only be the amount they paid for each session. After specifically adding their total payment due to reminder messages, I noticed more clients making it to sessions.

For example, one of my clients, a working mother of two, called at 4:30 P.M. to cancel her 5 P.M. session. She explained that she did not have childcare as her husband had to work late that day and would not be home in time to watch the children. After telling her exactly how much she would owe, the full ninety dollar session fee instead of her regular five dollar co-pay, within minutes she had called her housekeeper to stay with the children, allowing her to attend the session and avoid the full session fee.

For extremely unstable clients at high risk for negative reactions, you may wish to save your specific fee review to share at the beginning of the next session. By telling fragile clients in person instead of over the phone, you can more easily monitor their reactions and respond therapeutically to preserve rapport and treatment progress. As always, by staying calm and neutral in your words and demeanor, your clients are more likely to respond in kind.

Confidentiality

If someone other than the client answers your reminder calls, take steps to preserve confidentiality (see pp. 74–76). Ask to speak with clients directly and if they are not available, inquire when they will return. If you are told that clients will be back in about an hour, they are probably on their way to your appointment. If you are asked what the call is regarding, do not divulge your professional identity or refer to the services you provide. If you want to leave a message, keep it brief: "This is Jim Parsons. My number is _____, please tell him to return my call."

If you are comfortable sharing more, you can add "I'm calling about a 3 p.m. appointment today." Sometimes if you leave a short message a partner, roommate, or family member will know about the scheduled therapy and volunteer helpful information (e.g., the client is on his way to see you, he is out of town and must have forgotten, or any other reason for the late or missed appointment). They may also be able to reach the client faster than you could to remind him of the visit, and may offer to do so.

When my friend Dawn's client, Sara, did not show, she immediately called her to find out why. Sara was a young college student in therapy for test anxiety and as the semester progressed she had become more distressed. Sara's roommate, Mary, answered the reminder call and said that Sara was sleeping, having studied late the night before for an upcoming midterm. When Dawn shared the appointment, Mary immediately woke Sara up, helping her attend her much-needed therapy session and avoid a missed visit fee.

If you detect suspicion or negativity from anyone who answers your calls, do not share information or leave a message. Proceed to calling other available numbers to try and directly reach your client. You can also follow a general rule of not leaving messages with someone unless you know for certain they know about the therapy and the client has given you permission to talk with them. These days many people own and carry cellular phones wherever they go. By calling cellular numbers you have a good chance of directly reaching clients right away, avoiding confidentiality problems altogether.

My colleague, Frank, once narrowly avoided a disaster when making a reminder call to his client Maria, who was receiving individual therapy for depression and marital unhappiness. Maria's husband had refused to go to marriage counseling and was not aware that she had started therapy on her own. She described him as critical and controlling ever since they were together, which was a while since she had married at age 18 to escape an abusive father. The more steps Maria took toward independence, the worse things became in her marriage, but she was determined to be happy even if it meant eventually divorcing. Some of her therapy goals included building confidence and assertiveness, going back to school to get her college degree, and expanding her support network.

When Maria did not show for an appointment, Frank made his usual reminder call, forgetting that she had directed him to call her cellular phone and not her home phone. Her husband answered and angrily asked who Frank was and what he wanted. Quickly remembering her directive, Frank ended the conversation before sharing anything and was greatly relieved to have stopped in time to preserve confidentiality. He called Maria to alert her of the call so she could be ready if her husband pursued it further. Luckily he didn't.

Issue	Recommendation
Placing reminder calls to clients who do not appear for appointments.	1) To reduce no-shows, call clients after five or ten minutes as a reminder; use all available contact numbers and keep your professional identity private when leaving messages (pp. 183–184). 2) To facilitate attendance, review the policy and the specific missed appointment fee with clients during reminder calls (p. 184). 3) To preserve confidentiality when someone else answers reminder calls, ask for the client directly and do not divulge the purpose of the call (pp. 185–186).

Emergency Waiver

Another way you can be flexible with your policy is to waive cancellation fees for emergencies. If you do this, decide ahead of time which situations are severe enough to qualify as emergencies so you will have a guideline to follow later. Some scenarios will be obvious emergencies, like when my client Rebecca was rushed to the ER. However, many other situations clients present will not be so compelling or obvious. By setting your emergency criteria ahead of time, your task of enforcing the policy will be much easier when different events occur.

One emergency criterion you can use is an immediate physical injury or major trauma to the client. Typical examples include a hospitalization, involvement in a car accident, victim of a crime, serious illness/injury, and self-referral to urgent medical care. The same crises happening to one's children also qualify, given that the client is actively involved in securing help for the child.

For example, I received a call from a nurse at the emergency room of a local hospital. She shared that my new client, Amy, a woman in her 20s, who was scheduled to see me that day, had arrived with serious symptoms that turned out to be psychotic features of developing schizophrenia. Amy had remembered her appointment with me and told the nurse, who called right away. Although she was not hospitalized there, treatment was arranged in her home state and her family flew in immediately to help Amy move. This sad situation was definitely an emergency.

Another time my colleague Karen received a call from her client Victor, who was scheduled to see her the next hour. He explained that he had just been in an accident and was calling from a service station. Luckily Victor and the other driver were okay but his car was not—it was too damaged to drive. He had just called the police to report the accident and was planning to call his insurance company next. This immediate crisis was also an emergency.

When emergencies happen in your practice, if you offer clients a fee waiver, explain that this is a one-time exception to your policy and that they must call in advance to cancel appointments in the future. This will help reduce future missed visits by reminding clients that your cancellation policy is still in place. You can still reserve the option of allowing future emergency waivers based on individual situations and your own criteria. The following is an example of what you can say to clients after therapeutically responding to their immediate crisis needs:

> As you know, there is a twenty-four–hour cancellation policy and full fee required for the missed visit. However, because this is an emergency, I can waive the policy and fee this one time so there is no charge for this missed visit. However, for future sessions the policy will remain and you will need to call at least twenty-four hours in advance if you need to change your appointment. Would you like to schedule another session?

Non-Emergencies

You may find that many situations clients present at the last minute or after a no-show do not meet your emergency criteria. The following are some typical examples I have encountered:

1) (Two hours before the session) "Could I please change my appointment because I just remembered I have a gynecology appointment the same time as our session? It's the only one I could get so I would like to change our visit to another day."

2) (One hour before the session) "My boss just told me that I have to attend a mandatory work meeting so I can't come to my appointment. I'd like to reschedule, please."

3) (After not showing) "I couldn't come to my appointment because I didn't have any way to get there. My car is in the shop and my husband drove our only other car to work today."

4) (Six hours before the session) "I'm not feeling up to coming to my appointment today. I'd like to change it to another day.

None of these situations meets the criteria listed earlier to qualify as emergencies. In these and other non-emergency cases you can always follow your policy by charging the full fee for missed appointments.

When setting your own emergency guidelines you may choose broader or more restrictive criteria depending on the specifics of your practice (e.g., client populations, therapeutic specialty, work setting). You can also bypass this emergency waiver option completely and continue to follow the policy no matter what. My friend shared that this is what her therapist did. For every missed visit he charged clients the full fee regardless of the circumstances, whether an emergency or not. Whatever you decide, by developing your protocol in advance, you can more easily and quickly respond to situations when they do arise.

Issue	Recommendation
Waiving your cancellation policy for emergencies.	1) To determine situations that qualify for emergency fee waivers, develop your emergency policy criteria in advance (pp. 186–187). 2) To help set your criteria consider the following: immediate physical injury or major trauma to clients or their children, such as a hospitalization, an automobile accident, other serious illnesses or injuries, or being victimized by a crime (pp. 186–188). 3) To prevent future missed visits, present the emergency waiver of fees as a one-time exception to the cancellation policy (pp. 187–188).

Next-Day Sessions

Another way to amend your cancellation policy is to offer a substitute session later that day or within the next day or two. Clients receive a big break by not being charged for their missed appointment and treatment continuity is preserved. You also fill an open time that might otherwise go uncompensated. When offering this option, present it as a one-time courtesy to remind clients that the cancellation policy still applies for the future. You can also state the specific cancellation fee for added policy reinforcement.

Imagine that your client, Diana, calls right before her session to cancel, saying that she was just called to pick up her son from soccer practice early because he was in a fight. He wasn't hurt but was disciplined along with the other boy and told to go home. You could say, "Since there is the twenty-four–hour cancellation policy (and insurance doesn't pay for missed visits) your fee is $120. However, I do have an opening tomorrow afternoon at 3 P.M. If you are able to come to that appointment I can waive your cancellation fee."

If Diana can come to the appointment and tells you that she appreciates the fee break, you could respond with, "I'm glad we could reschedule your appointment this time, but if you cancel less than twenty-four hours again I cannot guarantee that I will have an opening. The cancellation policy will still be in effect and you would owe the full fee for the missed session. In your case the amount due would be $120 (since insurance will not pay for a missed visit)."

Phone Visits

If you reach clients on the phone during their scheduled appointment time, you can also offer a phone visit right then as a substitute for their missed session. Although clients will still be responsible for the no-show charge, this gives them the option to use their scheduled time as a phone visit. In the rare event that a client's insurance carrier pays for phone visits, you could also offer to waive the no-show fee and bill insurance for the phone session.

To prevent clients from assuming they can substitute a phone visit for a regular session whenever they want, present the offer as a one-time break: "Because there is the twenty-four–hour cancellation policy (and insurance doesn't pay for this missed visit), your fee is seventy dollars. However, if you'd like, you can have a phone visit right now to use the rest of your session time you are paying for with the $70. We wouldn't be able to do this in the future but if you'd like to I can make an exception in this case."

If new clients miss their first appointment, do not offer phone sessions to them. You haven't had the chance yet to evaluate them in person, establish a treatment plan, or obtain informed written consent. If you offer a phone visit without taking these steps you put yourself at risk therapeutically, ethically, legally, and financially.

One of my new clients, Scott, came to his first session after presenting over the phone with work stress and conflicts with his boss. During the inquiry call he made no mention of substance abuse. Throughout the interview Scott smelled strongly of alcohol, slurred his speech, had blood-shot eyes, and his clothes were disheveled. After questioning him more about substance abuse, Scott eventually admitted to a long history of drinking, DUIs, work absences, and was afraid of losing his current job. After much hesitation Scott agreed to go to an in-patient alcohol treatment program and I referred him right away.

If my first session with Scott had been a phone consult, there could have been a very different and disastrous result. It would have been easier for him to keep his addiction a secret and I would not have seen important non-verbal clues. Scott could have easily driven drunk again, hurting himself or someone else. At the very least, he wouldn't have been referred to the treatment he needed. The phone session would have unwittingly established me as Scott's treating clinician without full knowledge of the severity of his condition, a very dangerous position to be in.

Reduced Fees

Another option to have flexibility in your cancellation policy is to give clients a big break and offer a reduced fee (e.g., half of the full missed session charge). As with all breaks you offer, reinforce the policy and full fee for future missed sessions. In some situations you could also charge a fee smaller than half for missed sessions. For example, for insured clients who are responsible for a co-payment each session, you could accept this amount as payment in full for their first no-show.

Say that your client, Ted, does not show for his morning appointment. When you reach him that afternoon he tells you that he got his days mixed up and that he was planning to come tomorrow instead of today. He's been seeing you for quite some time and has been working hard in therapy to reduce severe social anxiety that he has struggled with all his life.

Because this is his first no-show you decide to offer him a break. When considering your options you cross off a substitute phone visit, as it's already past his appointment time. A next-day session won't work either because you have no available time the rest of the week. Finally, you decide to reduce his fee in half and say:

> Since there is the twenty-four–hour cancellation policy and insurance doesn't pay for this missed visit, your fee is eighty dollars. However, since this is your only missed session and you are very responsible, I would like to give you a break and charge just the half fee, or forty dollars, this time. However, if you do not make it to an appointment in the future and do not call twenty-four hours ahead to cancel, I'll need to follow the policy and charge you the full missed session fee of eighty dollars.

Payment Plans

An alternative option to a reduced fee is offering a payment plan to pay off any missed session charges. Clients receive flexibility in paying their bills and you preserve your original fee. This may work well with ongoing clients; they can make payments each session until they've paid their entire bill. For these reasons I usually offer this option instead of reduced fees to ongoing clients in my practice.

To avoid bending your policy too much, do not offer clients a payment plan for a fee you've already reduced. Since reduced fees are normally much smaller than your full fee, clients can typically afford to pay them at one time. In addition, do not offer payment plans for normal appointment charges; only consider them for missed session fees, otherwise clients may expect that they can spread out regular payments anytime they want.

To allow time to negotiate a customized plan in person with your client, offer the payment plan generally over the phone and wait to discuss it in detail at the next session. The payment frequency (e.g., weekly, bi-weekly) and amounts (e.g., ten dollars, twenty-five dollars) can be set up in many different ways depending on what is mutually acceptable. When discussing options, ask clients to share the payment plan that works best for them. By giving them control, you'll convey trust in their ability to set up and make payments. When clients are actively involved, they're likely to be more invested and follow through in honoring their commitments.

Instead of offering your client Ted a reduced fee, say that you decide on a payment plan instead. You could tell Ted, "Because there is the twenty-four–hour cancellation policy and insurance doesn't pay for this, your missed session fee is eighty dollars. I know you are very responsible and I'm sure we can work out some kind of payment plan to take care of this. Would you like to make another appointment now?"

Or, if you are concerned that Ted may react negatively upon hearing his exact fee owed given his severe anxiety, you could say, "Because there is the twenty-four–hour cancellation policy and insurance doesn't pay for this, you do have a missed session fee. I know you are very responsible and I'm sure we can work something out to take care of this. Would you like to make another appointment now?"

Assuming Ted sets another appointment, negotiate the payment plan with him at the beginning of his next session. For example, Ted's missed session fee is eighty dollars. He considers two forty-dollar, four twenty-dollar, or eight ten-dollar payments. He settles on two payments. Since he has insurance and his usual co-payment is twenty dollars, adding forty dollars brings his fee to sixty dollars for the next two sessions.

Issue	Recommendation
Offering substitute sessions and payment options to clients who miss sessions.	1) To waive cancellation fees, preserve treatment continuity, and fill open hours, offer clients substitute sessions available within the next two days (p. 189). 2) To allow clients who miss sessions to receive services during their scheduled hour, offer substitute phone visits at the full session fee (pp. 189–190). 3) To give clients a big financial break, offer a reduced fee for missed sessions as a one-time exception to your policy (pp. 190–191). 4) To provide clients flexibility in paying full missed session fees, offer a payment plan which they can create to pay off their bills (pp. 191–192).

CHAPTER NINE

Establishing Effective Phone Practices and Policies

When prospective clients inquire about your services, their first impression of you during phone contacts can determine whether or not they engage your services. If you've ever called someone for the first time and heard a stern, unfriendly greeting message, you know what a turn-off this can be. Or, imagine getting up the nerve to call for help and not hearing back for days. This chapter offers ways to avoid these and other pitfalls when responding to clients' inquiry calls. With careful attention to easily overlooked steps, you'll help clients feel comfortable asking for services and help ensure that they choose you as their therapist.

Sometimes ongoing clients seek unnecessary phone contacts between sessions. These calls can foster unhealthy dependencies, sabotage treatment goals, and become a major emotional and financial stressor for you. This chapter will also cover how to set up and implement a phone consult policy in your daily practice to help prevent these problems. By using your phone policy, you'll create effective therapeutic boundaries, preserve your time, and ensure payment for phone services you provide.

Employing Effective Phone Practices

Prospective callers are more likely to engage your services when you have ready access to a phone, check your messages often, and return inquiry calls right away. By conveying a positive demeanor in greeting messages and when making phone calls, you'll support clients in following through with the difficult task of asking for help. Maximizing the number of callers who become clients will allow you to reduce traditional marketing efforts, preserving your valuable time and funds.

Timing is Everything

When clients call the first time to ask about your services, at that moment they have decided to seek help. If you respond immediately there is a greater chance that they will follow through, as opposed to thinking it over and talking themselves out of it. For many people it has taken a while to gather the courage to ask for help and a quick response validates that not only is it okay to ask, but also that someone will be there for them when they do. By responding right away you show that you are available, attentive, and that you care. People are almost always in some level of distress when they seek help and will welcome concern demonstrated by a quick return call.

A potential client named Gene called my colleague, Susan, and she returned his call within minutes. He talked softly and sounded very sad, sharing that he had been recently diagnosed as HIV positive and didn't know how he was going to cope. He had been alienated from his family for years and his partner had died the previous year from AIDS. Although Gene had a network of friends, he had not told them about his status and was suffering alone.

By reaching him right away Susan was able to provide immediate support and encouragement, and he followed through in making an initial appointment. In the course of treatment Gene was able to tell his friends of his HIV status and accept their help, and he even started attending a local support group. He later shared with Susan that he was very ambivalent about calling for help, as he thought that any therapist would reject him just as his family had done. When she returned his call so quickly, he was very surprised and appreciative of her concern. He said that this made all the difference in his decision to pursue services, and in later asking for others' help, too.

Be the First Choice

When clients request services they often receive more than one clinician referral and will probably call various providers on their list at the same time. Multiple referrals occur frequently when people call their insurance carrier for names or look in provider directories. With the proliferation of Internet provider lists, clients are increasingly compiling their own referrals from this accessible information source. Clients may also ask their physicians or other professionals, who often give them three or more referrals from which to choose.

When you are one of many referrals, you will gain a time advantage and increase your chances of being the chosen therapist by returning calls quickly. This time factor is especially important when returning calls to clients with comprehensive insurance benefits, such as those provided through indemnity or PPO plans. These types of insurance usually do not restrict who clients can see or provide a large list of contracted providers. Because clients with these plans typically have a wider choice of clinicians than clients with other insurance plans (e.g., managed care), they are likely to call more therapists when initially seeking help.

Similarly, if clients present with common issues such as depression or anxiety, it's likely that many if not all considered therapists would be appropriate for the referrals. Because people may not tell you their insurance plan or therapy issues when leaving inquiry messages, by calling back right away you can find out whether you are a good match for their needs. If you do not return calls promptly or within an hour or two, these prospective clients are likely to connect with someone else first.

Think back to times you've attended professional workshops. During every break a majority of clinicians get right on the phone, busily listening to messages and returning calls. You can bet that some of these calls are to prospective clients, maybe even to the same people who call you to inquire about services.

Check Messages Often

An efficient communication system will help you receive and respond to calls right away (see Chapter 3). If you choose a messaging system such as a pager or cellular phone and carry it at all times, you will be immediately alerted when calls are received. Quickly check your messages and answer inquiry calls right away. To prevent call alerts from being obtrusive, set your system to vibrate instead of ring. If your system does not provide messaging alerts, routinely check for new messages throughout your day.

To identify inquiry calls to respond to immediately, do not directly answer calls; instead screen recorded messages as soon as you receive them. You'll save the time you would have spent answering calls that can wait, and make better use of those minutes to call back prospective clients. By using your time efficiently, you'll have a better chance of connecting with clients before they arrange for an appointment somewhere else.

During the hours you provide direct service to clients, check for new calls within your fifteen-minute breaks between sessions and return inquiry calls before starting the next appointment. If you see two or more clients in a row before returning these calls, with each hour that passes you are more likely to lose new referrals simply because you didn't call back sooner. Extend this habit of frequently checking messages when you are away from the office or performing other scheduled activities. Prospective clients will appreciate a quick return call and you'll increase your clientele with a minimum of effort. If you employ an outside answering service, receptionist, or someone else to make appointments for you, be sure she or he also prioritizes talking with prospective clients right away.

I use a pager as my messaging system and set it to vibrate mode, carrying it wherever I go. When the pager vibrates, I immediately listen to the voicemail message and return inquiry calls as soon as possible. During client sessions I tuck it inside my briefcase and pull it out to check for new message alerts in the fifteen-minute breaks between appointments. Because I sometimes see four or five clients in a row before an hour-long break, if I waited until the long break to call back I would probably lose many new referrals.

Use a Cellular Phone

To facilitate quick responses to prospective client calls, buy a cellular phone and carry it with you at all times (see Chapter 3). You'll have ready access to messages and you won't have to rely on finding a land line phone to return calls. You'll also be able to keep calls confidential by securing a private and quiet place to talk. With alternative public pay phones, you have no guarantee of privacy because other callers could stand next to you and you couldn't walk away in the middle of your call. If you are concerned about the cost, keep in mind that you can deduct cellular fees as a self-employed business expense. Also remember that by using your cellular phone, the benefit you'll receive of completing more client referrals will more than pay for the cost of the phone and service.

My former office neighbor, Joan, worked in many different locations. She ran groups at a hospital, made home visits through a hospice service, and saw clients in her private practice office. During a typical day, she was often in places where land line phones were not readily available (e.g., driving between jobs, at home visits, in groups). She used a pager as her messaging system and a cellular phone to place calls when away from the office or home. Because both were small and lightweight, she could easily carry them in her purse. When her pager went off, she was able to quickly access messages and return inquiry calls from her cellular phone from wherever she was at the time. For safety when driving, she always used a hands-free headset in the car. Although Joan's schedule frequently changed, her cellular phone allowed her to always remain available to new callers and assist them in making initial appointments.

Even if your weekly schedule does not vary, there will be times when you step out to run errands, attend appointments, pick up children from activities, take in an afternoon movie, have lunch with a friend, etc. If you don't have a cellular phone, you'll have to spend much more effort to find a land line phone to check messages and return calls. Although sometimes it may be challenging to find a private place for a call, the benefit of connecting with prospective clients is well worth the effort.

Once I searched many floors of a library for a suitable place to return a call and ended up in the women's restroom. Thankfully no one came in so I didn't have to leave before finishing the call. The caller was a young pregnant woman with three small children and full-time job responsibilities. Her husband had just died unexpectedly from a sudden illness and she was overwhelmed by the tragedy. She needed an appointment immediately and by calling back right away I could schedule her for a first available time. If I didn't have my cellular phone and had waited to call back, she may have connected with someone else first or suffered even longer waiting for help. She began individual therapy and later added family therapy with another therapist, eventually returning to work in a new routine for her and her children. Months after her husband's death she delivered a healthy baby boy and the entire family is continuing to heal, having ended therapy to continue on their own with help from family and friends.

In our line of work it gives pause to remember what major life traumas we work with and how the smallest things we do can be the most helpful. A simple step of carrying a cell phone and calling someone back right away may really help ease someone's suffering when they need it the most. You are also easily building your practice by being available and responsive at just the right time.

Issue	Recommendation
Responding to clients' inquiry calls.	1) To assist prospective callers in scheduling initial appointments with you, check for new messages often and return inquiry calls as soon as possible (pp. 193–195). 2) To identify priority inquiry calls, screen recorded messages upon receipt; to quickly return calls on busy days, call between sessions and/or at regular intervals (pp. 195–196). 3) To quickly review and respond to calls, use an efficient communication system and carry a cellular phone at all times (pp. 196–197).

Staying Positive During Client Contacts

Several practices will help you stay positive during client contacts. They include recording a positive greeting, using a caring tone, performing stress management regularly, and de-stressing your office.

Record a Positive Greeting

If you use a voicemail/answering system for calls, your greeting message offers clients their first and sometimes only impression of you. Many clinicians have their own messaging systems instead of a receptionist's service, so that prospective clients will probably hear a recorded greeting instead of a live person when they call. After contacting a few of these automated systems it can be frustrating for clients in distress to not be able to talk with someone right away. If your voice sounds distant or unapproachable, clients will be even more inclined to hang up as soon as they hear your greeting. In contrast, when your recorded message sounds kind and caring, it makes the uncomfortable process of leaving a message much easier for potential clients.

To create the best phone greeting, record your greeting as many times as needed until it sounds kind, supportive, and engaging. Do this anytime you change your message. For instance, if you need to change your greeting when you take trips out of town, review each new greeting to make sure it sounds helpful. After returning from a trip, you may be tired and your voice may convey this in your new greeting. Listen to your greeting the following day when you have more energy, and record the message again if needed until it reflects the positive qualities you want clients to hear.

If someone else answers your calls, their presentation is just as important and directly reflects on you. A person who comes across as interested and easy to talk with is much more likely to schedule new clients than someone whose demeanor is unfriendly. To ensure that your clients are receiving quality service, periodically ask for their impressions of phone contacts.

A clinician in my office building named Nancy used to pay an expensive answering service to take her calls. She had no idea that the receptionists were harsh, impatient, and unhelpful to callers. Only when her clients started telling her about their negative experiences did she realize how unprofessional the service really was. To make things worse, she didn't receive messages that clients said they left for her. Fortunately none of these calls were emergencies, but they easily could have been. Though Nancy called the service to complain, the problems continued as before. Fed up, Nancy switched to a much cheaper telephone line and pager, recorded her own greeting, and started taking her own calls. She now has complete control over the services clients receive and pays a fraction of the cost that the answering service charged.

Be Sure to Use a Caring Tone

When contacting clients directly over the phone, check to be sure that you are in a good state emotionally and not feeling extra stress at the moment you call. Your initial tone of voice and presentation can greatly influence whether prospective clients choose to see you or someone else. Many clients are survivors of emotional and other abuses and have a heightened sensitivity to any negativity, especially from an authority or caregiver figure. One small slip in the beginning could send clients fleeing to another therapist before even meeting you.

I've heard many people share that after talking to therapists during inquiry calls they decided not to pursue appointments. Although they typically gave some other reason for declining services, they secretly felt the therapist did not sound nice or easy to talk to. Although it's possible that the therapists were not nice, I'd guess they were having a stressful day, which can easily happen given the nature of our work. If these therapists had assessed their level of stress before returning calls, they could have taken steps to lower their stress or to remove the sound of it from their return calls.

Word Gets Around

Never underestimate how much clients can be affected by the smallest things you do and how often they may share with others the clinicians they like and those they don't. You probably expect clients to share these observations with friends and family, but they may also tell the referring parties who sent them to you in the first place (e.g., a fellow clinician, physician, or other referral source).

My colleague, Melanie, became acutely aware of this after one of her clients named Jessica shared that her referring physician, Dr. Kay, had been routinely asking for her feedback about Melanie's services. Jessica was severely depressed and anxious, a recovering alcoholic, and, a chronic smoker. To make things worse, she also suffered from hepatitis C, emphysema, and sciatica. She had grown up in a dysfunctional home with an alcoholic, abusive father and a codependent mother. Dr. Kay asked Jessica about her treatment with Melanie in every medical appointment, which was frequent given her poor physical condition. Jessica told Dr. Kay about her journal entries, letters she had written to her parents, stress and anger management strategies, her Adult Children of Alcoholics group, and so on. Dr. Kay was a very active and visible member of the community and had regular contact with many other physicians. If Jessica hadn't shared these inquiries, Melanie would have never known that Dr. Kay was so closely following her treatment.

Although not every referring party, family member, or friend may be so vigilant about your services, you can easily develop a negative reputation in a community without even knowing it. Although you keep details of your services confidential, your clients may not. Their impressions are like email messages; you never know where or when they will be forwarded. By keeping this in mind before client contacts, you can maximize your reputation and referrals and minimize the negative presentations you can't take back. Although Melanie's experience happened many years ago, Dr. Kay is still in practice and fortunately continues to refer clients to her.

De-Stress Before Returning Calls

To help maintain a positive and caring demeanor, de-stress before returning phone calls and anytime you need. When you are calm, pleasant, and attentive, clients will more often begin services with you as well as stay the entire course of therapy. Your positive reputation will grow as they tell others of their experiences and you will receive more new client referrals. You will also enjoy your work and stay healthy emotionally and physically. After investing many years in schooling and hard work, incorporating regular stress management will increase your practice longevity and years of earning power. In a profession vulnerable to burnout from stress, simple things you can do at work every day will help you to protect your-self and keep you viable. By extending these steps outside of work, you'll sustain and enhance these benefits wherever you are.

De-Stress Yourself

As practitioners we are very versed in stress management techniques and counsel clients all the time to use them. The main thing is to follow your own expert advice and incorporate these techniques into your own day. Often you'll be at your office when you need to reduce stress the most. If you have limited time, short strategies will work the best. Say you are between sessions and still feeling the stress from your previous hour of couples therapy when your client became furious after his wife divulged that she was having an affair. Although you are still shaken up inside, you check for new calls and listen to a potential client's inquiry message. You want to return the call before the next session, but you only have a minute to de-stress and regain a positive demeanor.

Before calling your prospective client, use one of your favorite quick de-stressors. You may prefer the 4-7-8 breathing technique, breathing in for four counts, holding for seven, and releasing for eight counts. If you are very rushed, you can take one deep abdominal breath. If you have a couple of minutes, consider a short, roundtrip walk, maybe to the restroom, down the hall, or up one flight of stairs. If you are concerned that you don't have the right shoes, keep a pair in your office for these quick jaunts. Maybe you'd rather stay in your office. You could sit or lie down for a quick meditation, focusing on a calming image or thought.

Perhaps you have more than a couple of minutes to de-stress. You could take a longer walk, going outside if possible. You'll receive rejuvenating benefits of light exposure and physical activity, even if your walk lasts just five or ten minutes. Or, you could call a colleague, partner, or friend to vent your frustrations and receive outside support. If no one is available you could journal to release stress. Maybe you have hobbies that would give your mind a rest. One clinician keeps a nerf basketball hoop over his wastebasket and pulls out his nerf ball for practice shots during breaks. Another takes her needlepoint project to the office, working on it a few minutes at a time. My former suitemate, Karen, relaxed by browsing through her catalogs for clothes, shoes, and home furnishings. Another colleague, Denise, enjoyed listening to her favorite Frank Sinatra songs on a CD player she kept in her office. I like listening to a five-minute relaxation tape I created that includes positive suggestions for working with clients. I keep it in a small recorder in my desk drawer so I can pull it out and listen to it anytime.

De-Stress Your Office

Simple steps, such as including pleasant lighting and furnishings can also turn your office into a calming environment. One fellow member of the group I joined kept a large aquarium in his office with many brightly colored fish. I remember feeling calm just sitting in his office, easily mesmerized by watching the fish quietly swimming in the background. Another group member in the office next door had a large collection of wind-up plastic toys on his desk. He used these to help bond with his children and adolescent clients. In addition, I think that everyone in the group had great fun watching the toys bounce up and down during breaks. Two of my current office neighbors use aromatherapy oils in their suites. I do, too, and many clients remark that as soon as they enter the office building they smell the calming fragrances. If you use certain therapeutic techniques during your sessions with clients, you may also benefit from their calming effects. I find when I've used hypnosis and EMDR with clients, I feel relaxed sometimes for hours after providing these interventions.

As you know, there are many additional stress reduction options and what you prefer might be very different. The important thing is to choose what works for you and build it in as a normal part of your workday. As therapists on the front line of delivery of care you can never give too much to yourself to restore the rapidly depleting resources you give to clients in need.

When Not to Return Calls Right Away

Once in a while your stress will be so high that these methods will not sufficiently release your tension. If so, wait until you are in a better emotional state before calling prospective clients back. For example, maybe you just had an argument over the phone with your partner, who was upset that you haven't been spending much time at home. Or, you could be feeling very irritable after having just finished a difficult client session. Perhaps the insurance company you just called was unable to fix an unpaid claim.

Sometimes only time will help to dissipate your stress to a reasonable level for a return call. By waiting to call potential clients back, you do run the risk that they will connect with someone else. However, if you call back feeling very stressed, your demeanor may put clients off and they could forgo services anyway. They may also tell others of their unpleasant experience.

One situation in which you should not wait to return calls is when potential clients call with immediate emergencies. In crisis calls, people will be so upset they probably won't notice your demeanor. They'll just remember that you were available to help right away.

Issue	Recommendation
Staying positive during client contacts.	1) To help clients feel comfortable in seeking help, record a caring and engaging greeting, reviewing and re-recording your message as needed (pp. 198–200). 2) To ensure that others who answer calls deliver positive, high-quality service, periodically survey your clients for their impressions of phone contacts (p. 199). 3) To ease clients' distress, enhance your reputation, and increase your practice longevity, perform stress management regularly and especially before contacting clients (pp. 200–203).

Employing Effective Phone Policies

One common stressor in private practice occurs when ongoing clients call between sessions to talk, but they are not experiencing a true emergency. These impromptu calls can interfere with clients' progress toward goals and harm therapeutic rapport. They can also be emotionally draining and time consuming for you, especially if you receive calls during personal time (e.g., nights and weekends). By setting phone call hours and informing clients of them at the beginning of services, you can prevent many of these potentially harmful situations. For clients who request and you agree would benefit, you could offer a phone consult between sessions. The following steps will guide you in creating your policy, introducing it to clients, and ensuring compensation for phone services you provide.

Phone Call Hours

By setting specific hours for routine calls, you can advise clients of your availability and set clear boundaries for contact. You'll help prevent clients from becoming upset if they call after hours and you don't call back right away. You'll also preserve your time and energy for your practice and private life. The therapeutic relationship is probably different from any other that your clients have experienced. They may not realize that you have boundaries unless you specifically tell them and clarify what to expect.

Therapeutic Benefits

Being clear about phone hours up front will help prevent clients from assuming that you'll be there whenever they need. This limit can be therapeutic for people who need to develop a support network. Instead of just relying on you, they'll be encouraged to reach out to others. During sessions you can reinforce this goal by helping clients identify steps they can take to connect with outside resources. You can also assist them in developing internal resources for times when no one is immediately available. Clients will become empowered and confident as they learn that they can take care of themselves.

My colleague, Sara, didn't identify phone call hours when she was new in practice. One new client, Debbie, called on Sara's day off sounding very distressed, and Sara returned the call right away. Debbie was a recovering alcoholic and although she had not been drinking, she angrily proceeded to review the many reasons she was upset with her husband. After unsuccessful and time-consuming attempts to calm Debbie, Sara said, "I need to go, but let's talk about this in our next session." After this exchange, Sara felt residual stress for quite some time, not a great way to spend her valuable day off.

When Debbie came to the next session Sara immediately reviewed her phone hours and the directive to call 911 in the event of a life-threatening emergency. Debbie appeared withdrawn and upset and Sara realized that by not specifying phone call hours or defining an emergency from the beginning, Debbie had not known the appropriate protocol. Sara had to spend effort and time to rebuild rapport, which delayed progress toward Debbie's original treatment goals.

To facilitate usage of outside resources, Sara recommended that Debbie attend daily AA meetings, meet at least weekly with her sponsor, and offered Debbie a referral to couples therapy. She also incorporated anger and stress management strategies that Debbie could use when no one was immediately available. After Sara specified this phone boundary, Debbie did not call to talk between sessions again. Instead, she called her sponsor and other AA friends. When she was alone she practiced her new self-calming skills. Now Sara specifies phone call hours and an emergency directive on her greeting message. She rarely receives calls between sessions from clients, and when they do leave messages, it's usually during her normal phone hours.

Announce Hours in Your Greeting

To inform clients of your phone call hours from the very beginning, state them in your greeting message. Anytime clients place calls, they'll be advised of your hours immediately. Potential clients calling for the first time, especially after hours, may feel calmer and more in control when they know the timeframe in which to expect return calls. Most new clients will probably call during business hours, so you're not likely to lose referrals by returning inquiry calls during set phone hours. The following is an example of a greeting you can use:

> Hello, this is Michael Owens, Licensed Professional Counselor. Please leave your confidential message including your name and phone number after the tone. Your call will be returned between 9 A.M. and 5 P.M. Monday through Friday. If this is a life-threatening emergency, hang up and call 911. Thank you for your call.

Clients are immediately informed that their call will be returned during usual business hours. They are also educated that an emergency is a life-threatening situation, and if this is occurring they should call the fastest, most equipped help via 911. Depending on your practice preferences, you could add or substitute a different instruction for clients to follow in emergencies. To ensure clients' safety, if they do leave messages stating emergencies, bypass phone hours and return calls right away.

Consider what Sara experienced—if you do not state your hours or define an emergency, clients are more likely to call anytime they feel an urgent need to talk. You'll have to establish boundaries after receiving calls, when you are probably irritated and at risk of reacting negatively. Your clients could perceive your new limit setting as punishment for something they didn't know was proscribed. Rapport could suffer and it may take time and effort to regain a positive working relationship. These problems are especially likely for clients with borderline, histrionic, or dependent personality features, whose trust and abandonment issues can be easily ignited.

If Clients Become Upset

Even when informing clients right away, someone may still become upset by your phone hours. However, if you keep returning routine phone calls after hours, your treatment will likely be compromised and you will be, too. The cumulative drain on your energy, time, and psyche is potentially more harmful to your practice than losing a client who perceives you as rigid and unavailable. If a client does stop services, you can offer the spot to someone else who is not upset by this boundary.

You'll probably find that most clients will accept your phone hours with no problem and the rare person who doesn't will likely end therapy early. Often people who drop out have seen many therapists in the past and present with clinically significant personality features (e.g., borderline or histrionic). These clients can be some of the most challenging and treatment resistant people to serve. A phone boundary can screen out these clients with a poor prognosis for improvement in traditional therapy, reserving your energy for people you have a good chance of helping.

When starting in practice I didn't state phone hours or define emergencies in my greeting message. Clients would call with urgent messages after hours, but when I called back it was almost never a true emergency. I quickly became frustrated at the amount of time and energy I was spending on unnecessary calls, especially after hours. I vividly remember one client, Gloria, who called late at night during an argument with her husband. When I returned her call, both Gloria and her husband got on the line using different phones, and their conflict continued with me in the middle. Although there was no physical violence or life-threatening emergency, this situation was extremely stressful and unsuited for a phone intervention. I also faced the foreboding task in the next session of addressing the episode, referring Gloria to marital therapy, and trying to discourage her from placing another destructive call.

Thankfully I eventually did add phone hours and emergency information to greetings. Since then the number of clients who call after hours has decreased dramatically. I suspect that most clients who do call are reminded of phone hours in the greeting message and hang up to turn elsewhere for immediate contact (e.g., friend, spouse, or family member). When people do leave a message, it's usually about canceling or changing their appointment and I return the calls during phone hours. If I had known when beginning in practice how much this information would deter after-hour calls, I would have added it to my greeting message before seeing my first client.

Tailor to Your Practice

When setting phone call hours and your phone consult policy, you may prefer different parameters from usual business hours. To help decide, assess features specific to your practice, such as client populations, work settings, and therapy specialties. Rely also on your training, experience, clinical judgment, and your comfort with the parameters. For example, my former suitemate, Denise, returns calls during her normal practice hours, from 11 a.m. to 8 p.m. This works well for her as the timeframe matches when she is at the office seeing clients. Some of her clients with severe depression and chronic pain appreciate being able to call in the evenings. They often sleep late and aren't fully functioning until late in the day.

Perhaps your practice is exclusively out-patient with average to high-functioning clients. If so, setting normal business hours for calls and consults may work fine. However, if many of your clients have complicated dual and multi-axis diagnoses, you may want to modify phone hours and consult options to fit your clients' needs. Maybe your therapy specialty is dissociative identity disorder and your therapy approach requires multiple phone contacts between in-person visits. Whatever phone policies you choose, by staying clear and consistent with your boundaries and fees, you will help clients honor the appropriate protocol in placing calls. You'll also preserve your treatment and practice viability.

Phone Consult Policy

If clients request phone contact between sessions and you agree that they would benefit, you could offer fee-for-service phone consultations during normal phone hours. Both self-pay and insured clients would typically be responsible for full charges because most insurance carriers do not pay for phone consultations. Although scheduling another in-person session for clients is preferable, there will be times when this is not feasible. For example, for insured clients you see weekly, many carriers will only pay for one mental health session per week. Other insurance plans have yearly caps; you may want to preserve sessions to ensure you have enough to complete treatment. Sometimes clients will be out of town or unable to attend the appointments you have available. Other clients may not request or require an entire therapy hour; a shorter contact may meet their needs.

When appropriate, offering phone consultations will reinforce the professional nature of your relationship and treatment. Unnecessary contact will be reduced as clients think twice before calling, deciding how important phone contact is based on the cost to them. The clients who do schedule consults will be more likely to value and respond to therapeutic interventions when they have invested their financial resources in this process. You will also ensure compensation for direct services you provide outside of regularly scheduled sessions.

Many other professions operate by billing for time rendered on the clients' behalf (e.g., attorneys, accountants, consultants), itemizing all tasks done for clients and billing accordingly. As mental health professionals we provide many services for our clients without direct reimbursement such as completing authorization requests, creating treatment plans and progress notes, billing insurance carriers, reading relevant literature, consulting colleagues, and making referrals. By charging clients for your time during phone consults, you can ensure compensation for this direct service and reduce unnecessary drains on your time, energy, and finances. This fee-for-service policy can be extended to other professional work that clients request that is not covered by third-party payers (e.g., specialized testing, assessments, and reports for other professionals).

For many years in practice I didn't have a phone consultation policy and didn't even consider creating one. By adding phone contact hours and emergency directives to my greeting, I was able to deter most after-hour calls. However, some people still called during weekdays asking seemingly brief questions—to verify their appointment time or to ask insurance questions. When I called back with answers, clients would typically bring up other issues that were often disruptive to therapeutic progress and goals. Other clients left urgent messages when there was no immediate crisis. These uncompensated calls grew lengthy and afterward I was emotionally drained.

I tried ways to limit these conversations in a kind but firm manner, but was always stressed after hanging up. Even the shorter calls became stressful, as I suspected clients were contacting me to the exclusion of other resources to help them get through the week. To reduce the frequency of these informal phone calls, I decided to set a phone consult policy and offer it to interested clients who would benefit. As soon as I started to tell clients who requested phone visits about this policy, the number of calls dropped radically. Now the few clients who pursue a phone consultation usually do not request another. Treatment is preserved and I save time and energy I would otherwise spend responding to unnecessary calls. When I do provide phone services, I am paid appropriately for my professional time.

Offering Phone Consults to Clients

To keep the number of phone consults you provide to a manageable limit, do not directly offer them to clients unless they specifically ask. If you wish, refer to phone consult fees in the new client form that clients complete in the first session. For example, the new client consent form in Appendix D states:

EMERGENCY PROCEDURES

If you need to contact me, leave a message according to the instructions on the phone service and your call will be returned. If an emergency situation arises, follow the emergency procedures and/or state that your call is an emergency. Please do this for true emergencies only. There may be a charge for lengthy telephone consultations.

If you predict that certain clients will call between sessions requesting phone contact, clarify the policy in person as early as possible. Often this will deter people from placing unnecessary calls and saves you the time and stress of responding to calls and explaining the policy over the phone. If someone calls before you explain the consult policy, for stable clients at low risk for negative reactions, explain the policy at that time over the phone. For fragile clients at high risk for reacting negatively, wait until the next session to discuss the policy. You'll be better able to respond therapeutically to unstable clients in person and minimize their distress in reaction to your policy.

Issue	Recommendation
Setting phone hours and offering phone consults.	1) To facilitate treatment and reduce unnecessary calls after hours, specify phone contact hours in your greeting message, tailored to your practice (pp. 203–207). 2) To reinforce the professional relationship, deter needless calls, and ensure payment for your services, offer fee-for-service phone consultations when appropriate to clients who inquire (pp. 207–208). 3) To keep phone consults manageable, do not directly offer them unless you are asked, except when you identify clients at high risk for placing calls (p. 209).

Phone Consult Hours and Fees

For clients who request, offer phone consults during your usual phone hours. This reinforces the professional nature of your contact and fits calls within your work hours, conserving the personal time you need to stay therapeutically effective and healthy. Quote specific phone consult fees based on each client's regular therapy fee, and inform clients that they are directly responsible for payment. On the rare occasion an insured client's policy pays for phone visits, share any co-payment responsibility.

Because insurance and fee-for-service rates can vary, calculating individual phone consult fees will ensure that you do not overcharge your clients. Compute fees before introducing the policy so you'll have specific numbers to quote. To simplify calculations, estimate charges based on a fifty-minute session. For example, based on a fifty-minute session fee of $100, a ten-minute phone consult is twenty dollars. By offering fees based on ten-minute increments, charges will be small enough to afford but large enough for clients to pause and consider whether a talk between visits is necessary.

The following is a typical introduction to a phone consult policy:

> I do offer phone consultations between sessions. If you are interested, we could set up a time to talk between 9 A.M. and 5 P.M. Monday through Friday. (Because insurance doesn't pay for this) I offer a prorated fee based on your regular session rate and how much time we talk. Since your fee is $100, if we talked for ten minutes your charge would be twenty dollars, twenty minutes would be forty dollars, and so on. Is this something you would like to do or would you rather wait to talk in our next appointment?

The Phone Consult

For clients who choose to proceed with a phone consult, schedule the day and time and estimate the length of the call. To give clients choice and control, offer two or more times that work within your schedule. To plan enough time and calculate consult fees, ask clients how long they would like to talk. Review fees and remind clients that they are responsible for payment. If you do not have a public number that clients can call for consults, place calls yourself and ask clients which number they'd like you to call. Confirm the day, time, fee, and number before ending the call.

The following is an example of what you might say when scheduling a consult:

I could talk with you Thursday at noon or Friday at 2 P.M. What time would work best for you? Okay, Thursday at noon will be fine. How long would you like to talk? Ten to twenty minutes sounds good. The charge will be from twenty to forty dollars, depending on how long we talk. What number would you like me to call? Okay, I'll call you this Thursday at noon at your home number. I look forward to talking with you then, goodbye.

During the phone consult write down the start and end time. Before finishing, confirm the day and time of the next therapy session and the exact consult fee due. To give clients a choice, offer options to send payment that day in the mail or to bring it to the next appointment. By collecting before or during the next therapy session, you'll reinforce clients' responsibility and follow-through in payment commitments. You'll also ensure timely payment:

Ok, so I'll look forward to seeing you at our next session this Wednesday, December 3rd at 3 P.M. We've talked for twenty minutes today so your fee is forty dollars. I know you are very responsible so you can either mail the payment to me today, or bring it to our Wednesday appointment along with your normal twenty-five dollar co-payment. Which would you like to do? Okay, so you'll bring the sixty-five dollars on Wednesday; cash or check (or credit card) will work fine. I'll see you then, Goodbye.

Privacy

If you will be home during consults, to preserve the privacy of your number, always place calls instead of receiving them. Although you'll pay for the calls, you can eventually deduct these payments as a phone business expense. Before placing calls from your home, call the phone company to have your number blocked, so clients and anyone else with caller ID will not receive your number (see Chapter 3, pp. 69–70). For added privacy, call the phone company to request that your home number be unlisted. Never give out your home number even if you believe clients will honor therapy boundaries. Once you share your number you have no control over who else might get it and clients or others they know may call at anytime.

Sometimes when placing calls you'll hear an automated message stating that the recipient does not accept blocked calls. Instead of unblocking your home number, switch to your cell phone and unblock it if necessary to make the call. Unless you use your cellular phone as your messaging system, remind clients at the end of the call to call your public work number for future contact (e.g., "If you need to contact me in the future, please call _____"). Clients will be discouraged from calling your cell phone even if they obtain the number through caller ID. To further deter calls to your cellular phone, do not set up voicemail or take incoming calls. If you do not want to restrict your cell phone to outgoing calls, call from your work or another public phone. For example, you could use a pay phone or a colleague's public phone. Whatever you choose, be sure to protect the privacy of your home phone.

Issue	Recommendation
Implementing effective phone consults.	1) To schedule efficient consults, offer times during usual phone hours, prorated fees, and review the day, time, number you will call, and estimated payment (pp. 210–211). 2) To reinforce clients' responsibility and follow-through in payment, offer options to mail consult fees that day or bring them to the following appointment (p. 211). 3) To protect your privacy when calling from home, block and unlist your home number; to reach clients who do not accept blocked calls, unblock your cellular phone and/or place calls from your work or other public phone (pp. 211–212).

Afterword

I wish you continued success as you consider incorporating these strategies into your unique plans for private practice. With increasing stressors such as violence around the world and where we live, we remain on the front lines providing services. The more stable and viable we can be emotionally and financially, the better we'll be able to provide quality care to our clients when they need it the most. I believe that economic uncertainties and hardships will become more dominant in the future with continued stressors such as job layoffs, roller coaster stock market rides, and personal/business bankruptcies. As potential clients are financially affected, they are more likely to forego fee for service therapy when basic expenses become a priority.

By using the streamlining strategies in this book, I believe that you will be able to see fewer clients and still earn a good living. You won't have to be frustrated investing more time and money marketing to a smaller pool of cash pay clients. You'll be able to provide service to clients with lower fee managed care insurance and remain financially viable. Whether you work part-time or full-time, see insured and/or cash pay clients, you'll protect yourself financially, even when the most unexpected occurs.

Appendices

APPENDIX A
Basic Expenses Estimation

Existing Expenses (#1)		
_____ Books	_____ Internet	_____ Auto
_____ Classes/ Seminars	_____ Business Calls	_____ Meals/ Entertainment
_____ Dues/ Subscriptions	_____ Postage	_____ Parking
_____ Supervision/ Consultation	_____ Supplies	_____ Travel
	_____ (_____)	_____ (_____)
_____ Total +	_____ Total +	_____ Total = _____ #1

Necessary Expenses (#2)	Recommended Expenses (#3)
_____ Professional License	_____ Medical Insurance
_____ Business License	_____ Disability Insurance
_____ Malpractice Insurance	_____ Life Insurance
_____ Continuing Education	_____ Accounting Services
_____ Total #2 +	_____ Total #3 = _____ #4

_____ #1 + _____ #4 = _____ #5 Total Monthly Basic Expenses

Note: Calculate monthly averages for each item.

APPENDIX B
Solo Expenses Estimation

Additional Start-Up Expenses (#6)	Examples
_____ Security Deposit	First and Last Month's Rent
_____ Furnishings	Furniture, Pictures, Plants
_____ Equipment	Fax, Copier, Computer, Printer
_____ Communications Systems	Phones/Set-Up Fees, Pager
_____ Billing (Option 1)	Computer Software
_____ Testing/Therapy Tools	WAIS-R, Play Therapy Toys
_____ Total #6	
Additional Ongoing Expenses (#7) Calculate monthly averages for each item.	Examples
_____ Rent	Monthly Rent
_____ Office Overhead Insurance	Quarterly or Yearly Payments
_____ Business Owner's Insurance	Quarterly or Yearly Payments
_____ Equipment Supplies/Repairs	Paper, Disks, Computer Repair
_____ Communications Fees	Monthly Calling Plans, Voicemail
_____ Billing (Option 2)	Monthly Services
_____ Other Supplies	Business Cards, Stationery, Forms
_____ Advertising	Yellow Pages, Internet, Publications
_____ Total #7 + _____ #5	Total Solo Expenses = _____ Monthly Expenses + _____ #6 Startup Expenses = _____ Grand Total Expenses

APPENDIX C
Benefit Check

Introduction and Network Status
This is _____, licensed (e.g., psychologist), and I am calling to receive (e.g., outpatient mental health) benefits for a new patient.   Note: The following questions are highly recommended for the first few times you call an insurance carrier; once you become familiar with each carrier's benefits you can skip many questions.   1. Is this an indemnity, PPO, EPO, POS, or HMO plan?   2. Does this plan require in-network providers?   3. Am I listed as an in-network provider?   4. (When you are not an in-network provider) Does this patient have out-of-network benefits?
Mental Health Benefits
5. What are the benefits?   6. Are you certain these are mental health and not general medical benefits?   7. Are you certain these are mental health benefits for non-MD providers? I am an (e.g., Ph.D.) licensed _____; will these benefits still apply?   8. Does this patient's insurance include parity benefits? (If yes) Could you please give me benefit quotes for both parity and non-parity diagnoses?
Benefit Maximums
6. How many visits are allowed each year?   7. What is the maximum dollar amount paid each year?   8. What benefits have already been used this year?   9. What is the lifetime maximum number of sessions?   10. What is the lifetime maximum amount paid?
Services Covered
11. Are any diagnoses excluded from payment (e.g., personality disorders, ADHD, conduct disorder, learning disorders)?   *Continued on following page*

219

Continued from prior page

12. Is (marital therapy) a covered benefit (provide a corresponding CPT code)? (other e.g., family therapy, testing, drug and alcohol treatment, hypnosis, EMDR)
13. (When applicable) This patient is also insured by another policy, is this insurance primary and should it be billed first?

Pre-Certification

14. Do visits require precertification?
15. Has precertification already been done for the patient to see me?
16. What is the approval number?
17. How many sessions have been approved?
18. What is the timeframe in which to use them?
19. What are the allowed CPT codes for these services?
20. Will a certification letter be sent to me?
21. What is the process to precertify?
22. What is the process to request future certifications?

Co-Payment

23. What is the patient's co-payment per session?
24. Does the co-payment increase as more visits are used?
25. What is the tiered co-payment schedule?
26. Does this co-payment schedule start over at the beginning of the year or any time during the year?

Deductible

27. Is there a deductible?
28. Does this deductible apply to both medical and mental health services?
29. How much is the deductible?
30. How much has already been paid?
31. Is this a calendar year deductible or does it start over at a different time in the year?
32 Are there any claims that have been recently submitted that will reduce the remaining deductible once they are processed?

Billing

33. What is the billing address to which to send mental health claims?
34. (If you are billing for out-of-network services) Is there a different address to send out-of-network claims?
35. What is the phone number for billing and claims?
36. Is there a special claim form required for billing or can I use the standard CMS (HCFA)-1500 claim form?

APPENDIX D
New Client Form

(Your Letterhead)

Welcome to my practice. I look forward to helping you reach your goals. This form requests information about your needs and informs you of my services and policies. Please take a few moments to complete this form. The questions on the following pages are designed to help me best meet your treatment needs. If the person seeking care is a child, the parent or guardian should complete this form. If you have any questions, I will be happy to answer them.

Client Name _____ Birthdate _____

Address _____ Age _____

City, State, Zip _____ Gender ☐ Female ☐ Male

Client SSN _____ Relationship Status Single Married Domestic Partner
                                                     Separated Divorced Widowed

Mental Health Plan _____ Full Time Student? ☐ Yes ☐ No

Medical Health Plan_____ Occupation _____

Primary Care Physician _____ (____) _____
                                                           Phone

Your Phone # (____) _____ (____) _____
            Home   OK to contact there? Y N   Work   OK to contact there? Y N

Emergency Contact_____ (____) _____
                     Name   Relationship to client   Phone number

Please list other persons living in your household and their relationship to you:

_____

_____

Primary Insurance Information	Secondary Insurance Information
Insured Name _____	Insured Name _____
Insured SSN _____	Insured SSN _____
Insured Birthdate _____	Insured Birthdate _____
Employer _____	Employer _____
Payer/Health Plan_____	Payer/Health Plan _____
Client's Relationship to the Insured:	Client's Relationship to the Insured:
☐ Self ☐ Spouse ☐ Dependent	☐ Self ☐ Spouse ☐ Dependent
Member # _____	Member # _____
Policy/Group # _____	Policy/Group # _____

Continued on following page

Continued from prior page

1. Please describe your reason(s) for seeking treatment at this time. If there is a particular event which triggered your decision to seek treatment now, please list the event:

_____

_____

_____

2. Please indicate how the issue(s) for which you are seeking treatment are affecting the following areas of your life:

	No effect	Little effect	Some effect	Much effect	Significant effect	Not Applicable
Marriage/Relationship	1	2	3	4	5	N/A
Family	1	2	3	4	5	N/A
Job/School performance	1	2	3	4	5	N/A
Friendships	1	2	3	4	5	N/A
Financial situation	1	2	3	4	5	N/A
Physical health	1	2	3	4	5	N/A
Anxiety level/Nerves	1	2	3	4	5	N/A
Mood	1	2	3	4	5	N/A
Eating habits	1	2	3	4	5	N/A
Sleeping habits	1	2	3	4	5	N/A
Sexual functioning	1	2	3	4	5	N/A
Alcohol/Drug usage	1	2	3	4	5	N/A
Ability to concentrate	1	2	3	4	5	N/A
Ability to control your temper	1	2	3	4	5	N/A

3. What result(s) do you expect from treatment?

_____

_____

4. Have you ever received mental health treatment before? If so, please list dates, provider name, and the issue for which treatment was sought:

_____

_____

5. Please list any medications you're currently taking:

_____

_____

TREATMENT PHILOSOPHY
I believe in providing goal-directed treatment. This means that a treatment goal or several goals are established after a thorough assessment. All treatment is then planned with the goal in mind and progress is made toward accomplishment of that goal in a time-efficient manner. If you ever have any questions about the nature of the treatment or anything else about your care, please don't hesitate to ask.

CONFIDENTIALITY
All information between provider and patient is held strictly confidential unless:

1. The client authorizes release of information with his/her signature.
2. The client presents a physical danger to self.
3. The client presents a danger to others.
4. Child/elder abuse/neglect are suspected.

In the latter two cases, I am required by law to inform potential victims and legal authorities so that protective measures can be taken.

FINANCIAL TERMS
Upon verification of health plan/insurance coverage and policy limits, your insurance carrier will be billed for you and I will be paid directly by the carrier. You will be responsible for any applicable deductibles and co-payments. Co-payments must be paid at the time services are rendered. If you are not eligible at the time services are rendered, you are responsible for full payment.

CANCELLED/MISSED APPOINTMENTS
A scheduled appointment means that time is reserved only for you. If an appointment is missed or cancelled with less than twenty-four–hours notice, you will be billed directly according to the scheduled fee or according to the rules of your health plan. Your health plan does not cover payment for missed appointments; therefore, you are responsible for payment in full.

EMERGENCY PROCEDURES
If you need to contact me, leave a message according to the instructions on the phone service and your call will be returned. If an emergency situation arises, follow the emergency procedures and/or state that your call is an emergency. Please do this for true emergencies only. There may be a charge for lengthy telephone consultations.

RELEASE OF INFORMATION
I authorize the release of information regarding my care to my health plan for the payment of claims, certifications/case management decisions, and other purposes related to the administration of benefits for my health plan.

CONSENT FOR TREATMENT
I further authorize and request that my treating provider carry out mental health examinations, treatments, and/or diagnostic procedures, which now or during the course of my care are advisable. I understand that the purpose of these procedures will be explained to me upon my request and subject to my agreement. I also understand that while the course of therapy is designed to be helpful, it may at times be difficult and uncomfortable.

I understand and agree to all of the above information.

_____   _____
Client (or Parent/Guardian) Name—Printed   Date

_____   _____
Client (or Parent/Guardian) Name—Signature   Date

APPENDIX E
Billing/Practice Tasks Checklist

Daily	Weekly
Between Sessions	At the End of the Client Week
Client-Oriented Tasks	**Billing Tasks**
_____ Return urgent/inquiry calls	_____ Close and print log report
_____ Type the session's progress note	_____ Print claims and mailing labels
_____ Prepare for the next session	_____ Sign claims with signature stamp
Billing Tasks	_____ Sort and mail claims
_____ Record your service	_____ Back up data
_____ Record the client's payment	_____ Do virus protection/firewall update
	_____ Fix incorrect insurance payments
During Other Available Time	During Any Available Time
Billing Tasks	**Other Tasks**
_____ Create new client files	_____ Complete authorization requests
_____ Record insurance payments	_____ Type reports/correspondence
_____ Conduct benefit checks	_____ Consult with colleagues
_____ Record new authorizations	_____ Read professional publications
Other Tasks	_____ Pay bills
_____ Return non-client calls	_____ Purchase supplies as needed
_____ File progress notes	
_____ Read mail	

Bi-weekly or Monthly
Billing Tasks
_____ Generate outstanding insurance reports
_____ Call insurance carriers to facilitate unpaid claims

APPENDIX F
Financial Tasks Checklist

Weekly	Monthly
Preparing Deposits	**Preparing Financial Reports**
_____ Fill out deposit slip	_____ Reconcile account upon receiving monthly bank statement
_____ Copy deposit slip and payments	_____ Print reconciliation summary
_____ Endorse checks with deposit stamp	_____ Print transaction report (e.g., Jan. 1–31)
_____ Prepare deposit envelope	_____ Total cash payments/mileage record
_____ Place ATM deposit that day	_____ File bank, reconciliation, transaction, cash payments, and mileage reports
_____ Record deposit in checkbook register and computer program	_____ (File practice log reports weekly)

Quarterly
Sending Financial Reports
_____ Send bank, reconciliations, transaction, cash payments, mileage, and log reports to accountant

APPENDIX G
Professional Organizations

American Association for Marriage and Family Therapy
112 S. Alfred St.
Alexandria, VA 22314
(703) 838-9808
www.aamft.org

American Counseling Association
5999 Stevenson Ave.
Alexandria, VA 22304
(800) 347-6647
www.counseling.org

American Mental Health Counselors Association
801 N. Fairfax St., Ste. 304
Alexandria, VA 22314
(800) 326-2642
www.amhca.org

American Psychiatric Association
1000 Wilson Blvd., Ste. 1825
Arlington, VA 22209-3901
(703) 907-7300
www.psych.org

American Psychological Association
750 First St., NE
Washington, DC 20002-4242
(202) 336-5500
www.apa.org

National Association of Social Workers
750 First St., NE, Ste. 700
Washington, DC 20002-4241
(202) 408-8600
www.socialworkers.org

APPENDIX H
Additional Practice Management Resources

Building Your Ideal Private Practice: A Guide for Therapists and Other Healing Professionals, by Lynn Grodzki. W.W. Norton & Company, 2000.

Business Strategies for a Caring Profession: A Practitioner's Guidebook, by Sharon L. Yenney. American Psychological Association, 1994.

Getting Started in Private Practice, by Chris E. Stout. John Wiley & Sons, 2004.

How to Build a Thriving Fee-For-Service Practice: Integrating the Healing Side with the Business Side of Psychotherapy, by Laurie Kolt. Academic Press, 1999.

Independent Practice for the Mental Health Professional: Growing a Private Practice for the 21st Century, by Ralph H. Earle and Dorothy J. Barnes. Brunner/Mazel, 1999.

The Paper Office: Forms, Guidelines and Resources (3rd ed.), by Edward L. Zuckerman. Guilford Press, 2003.

The Psychotherapist's Guide to Managed Care in the 21st Century: Surviving Big Brother and Providing Quality Mental Health Services, by Sondra Tuckfelt, Jeri Fink, and Muriel Prince Warren. Jason Aronson, 1997.

Psychotherapy Finances, newsletter published monthly for mental health providers. Call (561) 748-7816, www.psyfin.com

Saying Good-Bye to Managed Care: Building Your Independent Psychotherapy Practice, by Sandra Haber, Elaine Rodino, and Iris Lipner. Springer Publishing Company, 2001.

Successful Private Practice: Winning Strategies for Mental Health Professionals, by Susan Frager. John Wiley & Sons, 2000.

Twelve Months to Your Ideal Private Practice: A Workbook, by Lynn Grodzki. W.W. Norton & Company, 2003.

Index

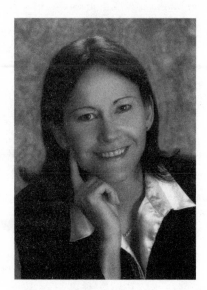

Holly A. Hunt, Ph.D., is a psychologist in private practice in Southern California, where she first established her practice in 1990. She received her Ph.D. in Clinical Psychology from the University of Kansas in 1988. Hunt interned at the VA Medical Center in Sepulveda, California and then worked as a staff psychologist at the VA Medical Center in Long Beach. She is the past Chair of the Practice Management Committee of the San Diego Psychological Association. Hunt provides workshops on the topic of establishing and maintaining a streamlined private practice.

For additional information, speaking on related topics, and/or personal consultation regarding your practice, contact:

Holly A. Hunt, Ph.D.
5855 E. Naples Plaza, Ste. 309
Long Beach, CA 90803
(562) 987-8947
www.EssentialsOfPrivatePractice.com

Photo credit: Martin Mann